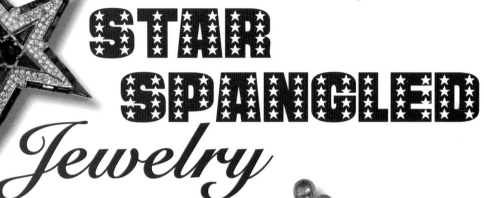

STAR SPANGLED Jewelry

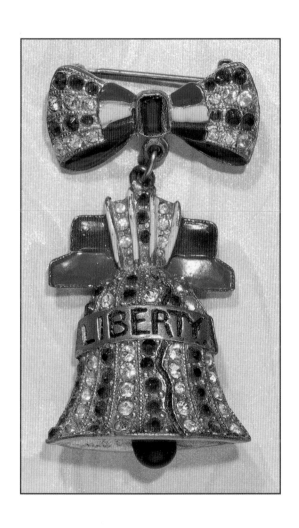

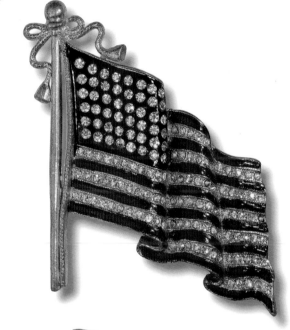

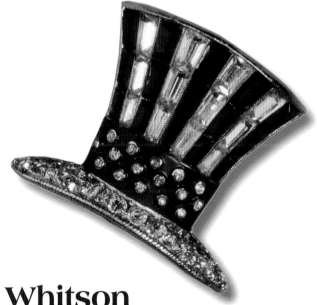

Sandra J. Whitson
with Nancy N. Schiffer

Dedication

This book is dedicated to the memories of both my Dad
Frank G. Whitson
and my sister
Elizabeth Scheuerman.
They added so much sparkle to my life!

The items shown in the following photographs are from the collection of Sandra J. Whitson and are vintage, 1920-1970, unless otherwise noted.

Other Schiffer Books on Related Subjects:
Sweetheart Jewelry and Collectibles Nick Snider
Antique Sweetheart Jewelry Nick Snider

Copyright © 2007 by Sandra J. Whitson and Schiffer Publishing Ltd.
Library of Congress Control Number: 2007920059

Designed by John P. Cheek
Cover design by Bruce Waters
Type set in Americana XBd BT/Zurich BT

ISBN: 978-0-7643-2648-6
Printed in China

Published by Schiffer Publishing Ltd.
4880 Lower Valley Road
Atglen, PA 19310
Phone: (610) 593-1777; Fax: (610) 593-2002
E-mail: Info@schifferbooks.com

For the largest selection of fine reference books on this and related subjects, please visit our web site at
www.schifferbooks.com
We are always looking for people to write books on new and related subjects. If you have an idea for a book please contact us at the above address.

This book may be purchased from the publisher.
Include $3.95 for shipping.
Please try your bookstore first.
You may write for a free catalog.

In Europe, Schiffer books are distributed by
Bushwood Books
6 Marksbury Ave.
Kew Gardens
Surrey TW9 4JF England
Phone: 44 (0) 20 8392-8585;
Fax: 44 (0) 20 8392-9876
E-mail: info@bushwoodbooks.co.uk
Website: www.bushwoodbooks.co.uk
Free postage in the U.K., Europe; air mail at cost.

Contents

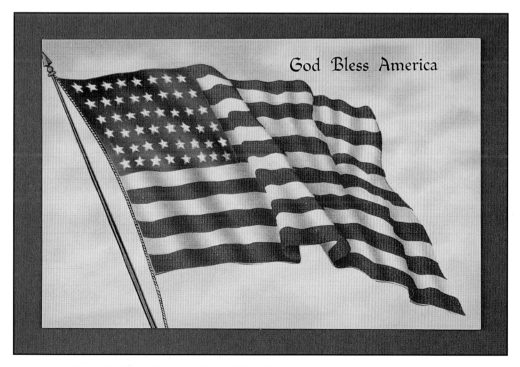

Postcard, 1941. "Tichnor Quality Views" Flag Series No. 1.

Acknowledgments

While the vast majority of the pieces shown in this book are from the collection of the author, there are a number of people to thank for their assistance and willingness to share as the book was being formulated.

The only other person who loaned items from her collection to be photographed was Barbara Trujillo, from Bridgehampton, New York. Barbara's enthusiasm and love for the patriotic jewelry definitely rivals mine. She is a joy to be around.

One of my mentors, in my early collecting years, was Richard Silverman. His knowledge of costume jewelry exceeds the ordinary and he has always been very generous in sharing information and finding me some great pieces. I remember many days with him at Brimfield, Massachusetts, when my Dad called Richard and his brother "the rhinestone cowboys."

Another early influence was Dorothy Bauer, whose company is today Dorothy Bauer Designs. In 1982, her fledgling company was called A Piece of the Rainbow and I was buying wonderful designs from her.

Jackie Fleischmann is a dear friend who is also extremely knowledgeable about costume jewelry. Life has not always dealt Jackie an easy hand, but she remains cheerful and always ready to help others. When I first started collecting, Jackie sold two wonderful flag pins to my Dad for me.

Kenneth Sheldon is an antiques dealer who specializes in costume (and other) jewelry. Ken has found me some outstanding pieces of jewelry that I am proud to have in my collection.

A special thanks goes to Karl Eisenberg, who runs the Eisenberg empire started by his grandfather, and to Bobye Syverson, of Bobye's Enchanted Castle, in Wisconsin. Both of them were very helpful in supplying information about Eisenberg jewelry.

Another contributor, who didn't even know that he was contributing to my book, is Stuart Weitzman, the genius shoe designer who created my wonderful flag shoes and purse from his Pavé Collection.

My appreciation is extended to Steve and Linda Sherwin for the beautiful etched flag wine bottle, which is exquisite. Also, thanks to my friend, Carol Cali, who was so instrumental in getting me together with the Sherwins.

Doug Congdon-Martin and Bruce Waters did an outstanding job with the photography for the book; it was a joy to work with them. Last, but not least, a giant thank you to Nancy Schiffer. The book would never have been completed without her.

To all of the above and any I have inadvertently omitted, I am most grateful.

Sandra J. Whitson

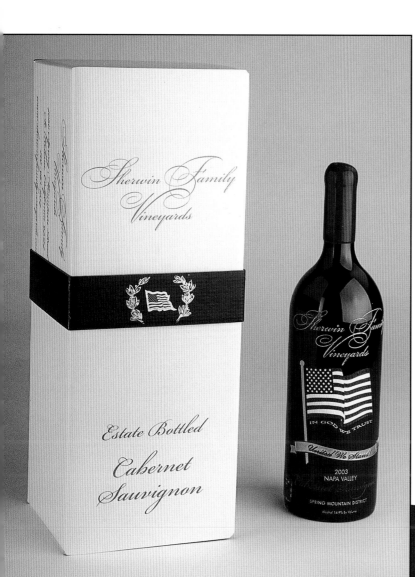

Commemorative wine bottle with etched and hand painted American flag
Sherwin Family Vineyards, St. Helena, California
Steve and Linda Sherwin
Courtesy of Sherwin Family Vineyards

After the terrorist tragedies of September 11, 2001, there was a wine auction in Garda, Italy, to benefit the families of the tragedy. Fifty Napa Valley, California, wineries sent wine to Italy, where they were each paired with an Italian wine for the auction. Steve and Linda Sherwin, of Sherwin Family Vineyards, wanted to "dress-up" their bottle to meet the occasion. They had the American flag etched and hand painted, with a tribute on the back, to the families of the people who died in the Windows on the World restaurant at the top of the World Trade Center in New York. After the auction, Steve and Linda were so pleased with the results that they decided to produce more of the commemorative flag bottles for future charity events and private sales for collectors. After many hours of telephone calls and research, the American Flag bottle finally made its way to Washington, D.C., where it received its stamp of approval. As known, this is the first and only alcohol bottle ever approved to bear the American Flag for legal sale. Upon receiving the bottle, various United States presidents and senators have been so touched that they have taken the time to personally call and thank the Sherwin Family. The flag is only placed on large format bottles; they are numbered and only sold through their winery.

Above: A letter of thanks signed by William H. Frist, M. D., March 25, 2004. Below: A letter of thanks signed by George W. Bush, October 21, 2002.

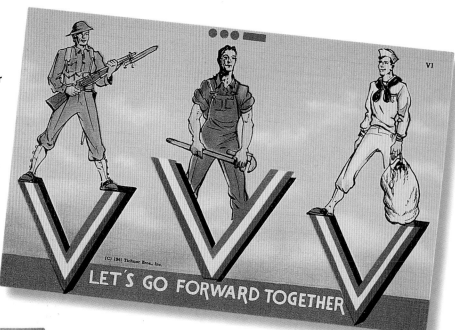

Postcard, 1941. "Tichnor Quality Views" Victory Series No. 1.

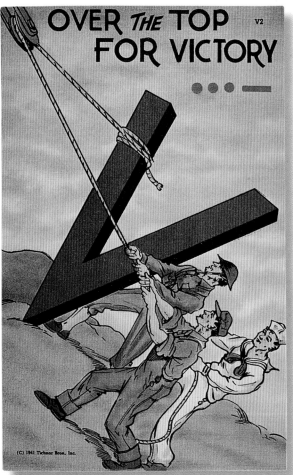

Postcard, 1941. "Tichnor Quality Views" Victory Series No. 2.

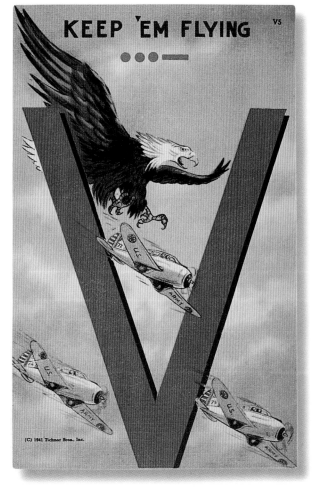

Postcard, 1941. "Tichnor Quality Views" Victory Series No. 5.

Introducing Patriotic Jewelry

Rhinestone jewelry, once so popular, then rejected as cheap and gaudy, is back in vogue! It is being sold in many stores and you cannot turn on the television or watch a movie without seeing a vast array of sparking rhinestone jewelry. It is a regular practice for politicians and spouses of politicians to wear rhinestone American flag pins proudly. Yet, the older pieces have become a much sought-after collectible. You may see some high prices on rhinestone, or costume, jewelry in antique shows, especially in larger, metropolitan cities, but this is a category of accessories that is still affordable and fun.

Costume jewelry has been around for a very long time. In the Depression era of the 1930's, women who could not afford a new dress could find an inexpensive costume jewelry piece to change the look of an old dress and lift their spirits. As Maryanne Dolan wrote in her book, *Collecting Rhinestone Jewelry,* "Life was dark and rhinestones were bright." In the 1930s and 1940s, different levels of this affordable jewelry could be purchased at both an elegant jewelry store and the corner 5-and-dime.

A very special niche of rhinestone jewelry has United States patriotic significance. Whereas this jewelry was being created during the First World War, it was in the 1940s that patriotism was running at a fever pitch. As the United States was becoming more involved in World War II, wearing patriotic pins gave people at home something with which to honor their loved ones in service at home and abroad, while also showing patriotism for their country.

There was another influx of United States political jewelry in the 1950s. Members of national women's society The Daughters of The American Revolution sold little rhinestone flag pins to raise money for their organization. Again in 1976, which marked the American Bicentennial birthday, patriotic styles were often worn and displayed proudly. More recently, the tragedy of September 11, 2001 caused American flags to be flown everywhere in the world for remembrance and support of the grieving families. Everyone wanted to wear a patriotic pin to show unity with the United States. There were no Democrats or Republicans then, just Americans showing their support for the country they love.

Many books about costume jewelry present details about the manufacturers and the processes of making rhinestone jewelry, and some are sited in the Bibliography. Some people put a lot of emphasis on "signed" costume jewelry (i.e., bearing a company trademark or signature). Often, those pieces do command higher prices. Yet, there are some outstanding early flags and other jewelry that were never signed. The quality and rarity of those pieces speak for themselves. Some of the favorite pieces in my collection are not signed.

This book is intended to be fun. It is by no means all-inclusive regarding the scope of what was created in this field. There seems to be an endless supply of vintage patriotic jewelry and other patriotic pieces, so go out and enjoy finding them. I hope only to whet your appetite by showing the vast array of types that can be found in the patriotic world. The excitement that this jewelry creates is contagious. Whether you are buying it for fun, investment, or to celebrate a portion of history, you can enjoy the aura and appreciate the heritage behind this sparkling bit of Americana.

Flags

No symbol evokes such strong feelings of patriotism and loyalty to the United States as the American flag. On June 14, 1777 (the first "Flag Day"), a flag, of 13 stripes alternating red and white, and 13 stars on a blue field, was adopted to signify the new country, The United States of America. I am of the generation that was taught that Betsy Ross made the first stars and stripes flag. Whereas most historians today reject this as untrue; the story is still a wonderful part of American folklore.

When Francis Scott Key saw the American flag flying over Fort McHenry in Baltimore, Maryland, on the morning of September 13, 1812, after British bombardment that had continued for 25 hours, he penned the poem that later became the National Anthem.

In a 1945 battle during the Second World War at Iwo Jima, United States Marines raised the American flag and were photographed for a now-famous image that nearly everyone recognizes today. It evokes the hardship of securing national principles and the thrill of military victory. It is an image that brings pride to all Americans.

When United States astronauts landed on the moon in 1969, the American flag was planted there to signify a civilian victory over the unknown place. That accomplishment continues to give people pride in America.

After the tragedy of 9/11/01, raising the American flag at the site of the World Trade Center in New York recalled memories of the flag raised at Iwo Jima.

Through celebratory times and through tragic times, the American flag has brought hope, unity, and promise to many people around the world and especially in the United States of America.

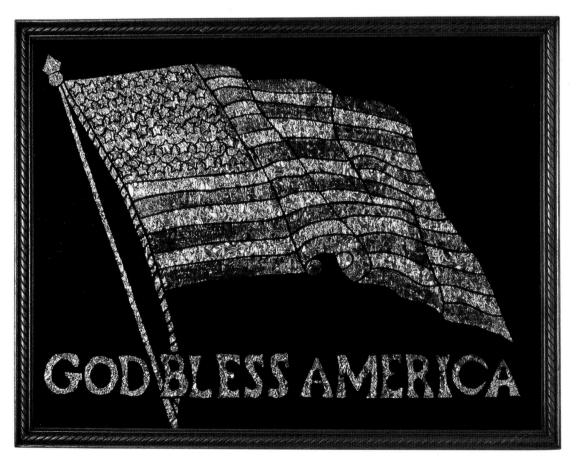

Glass picture in a frame, decorated from the back with foiled American flag and "God Bless America." 17" x 13". Unmarked. 1970s.

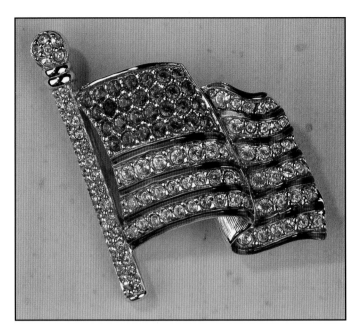

Waving American flag pin with Swarovski crystals. Unsigned. Contemporary.

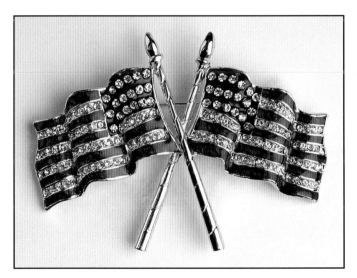

Pin of crossing American flags in gold metal with enamel and clear rhinestones, 2-1-4" wide. Contemporary.

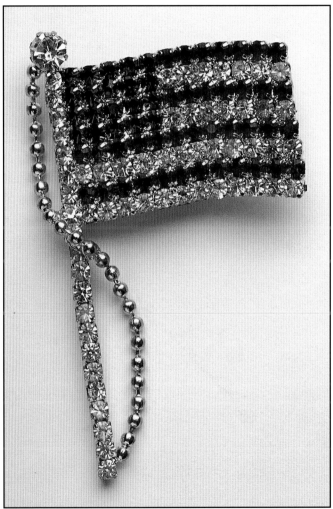

Flag pin with gold ball chain and red, white, and blue rhinestones. Contemporary.

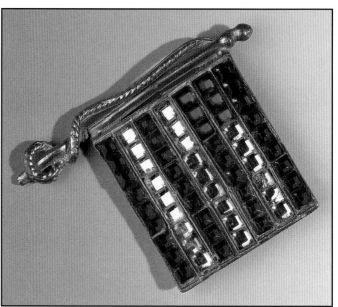

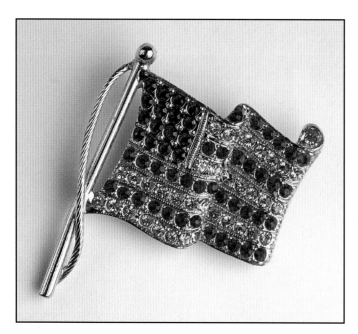

Flag pin of gold metal with red, white, and blue rhinestones. Contemporary.

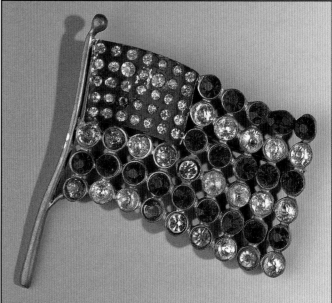

American flag pin with red and clear rhinestones. Courtesy of Barbara Trujillo.

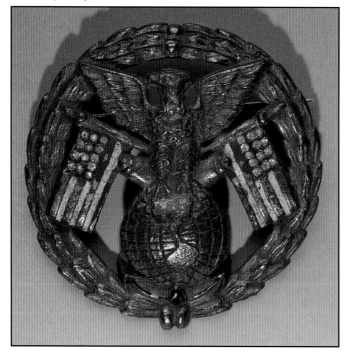

Eagle sitting atop the globe and American flags on either side. Courtesy of Barbara Trujillo.

Pin with eagle sitting in the center of a "V" and American flags on either side. Courtesy of Barbara Trujillo.

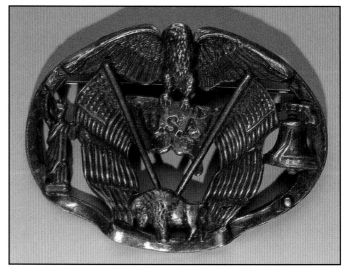

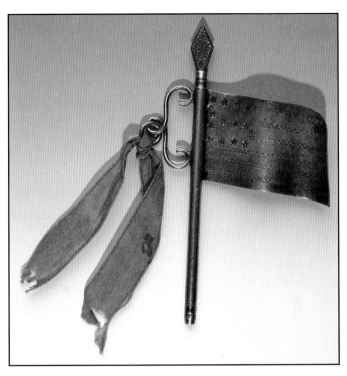

American flag with banner. Courtesy of Barbara Trujillo.

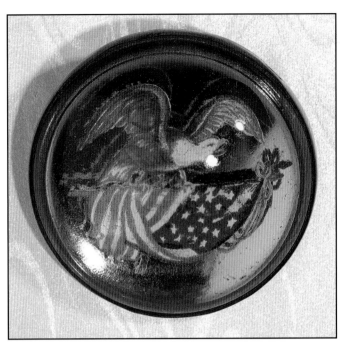

Pin with eagle carrying the American flag. Bridle button. 1970s.

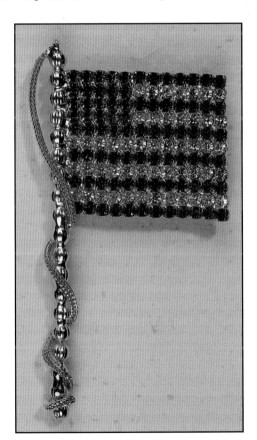

Gold American flag pin. 3 5-8" tall. Signed "Dominique". 1992.

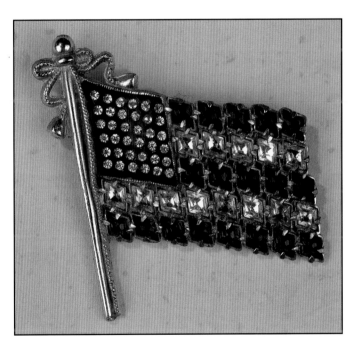

Large American flag pin with red and clear diamond shaped rhinestones. 2 1-4" x 2 1-2". Unsigned. WWII period.

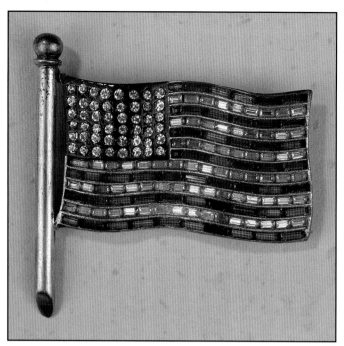

Beautiful American flag pin in red, blue, and clear rhinestones. By Ciner. 2" wide. WWII period.

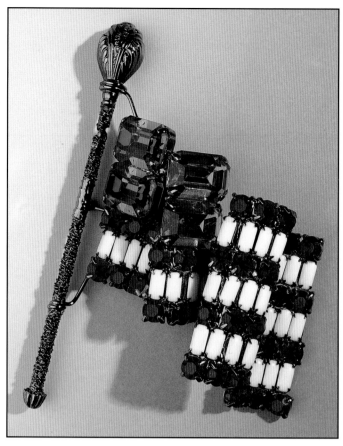

Fabulous large flag pole pin with American flag in rhinestones and milkglass with a wide, huge furl. Flag pole is 4 3-8" tall. Flag is 2 1-2". By Lawrence Vrba, contemporary designer.

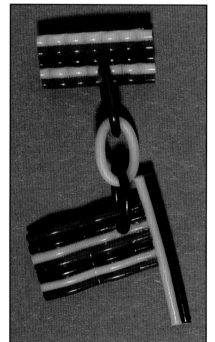

Celluloid American flag in red, white, and blue colors, dangling from a bar pin. 1940s.

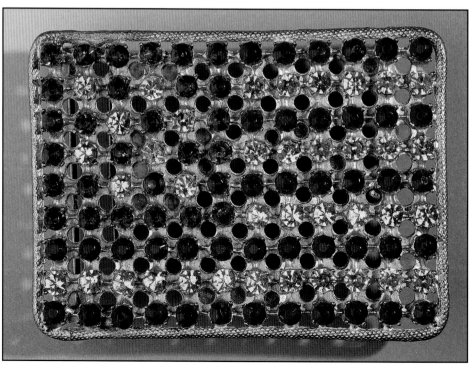

American flag belt buckle. 3" x 2 1-8".

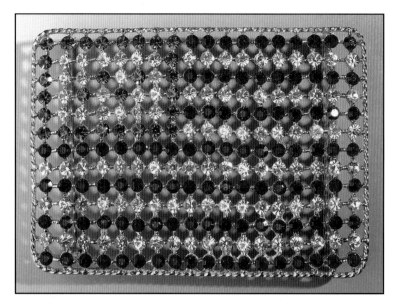

American flag belt buckle. 4 3-8" x 3 1-4".

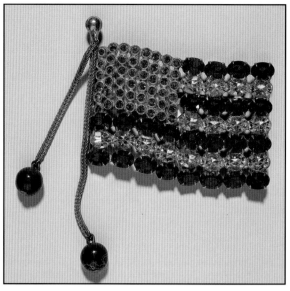

American flag pin of large red and clear oval faceted rhinestones and blue collet-set small stones. Two gold mesh ropes with red beads. Unmarked. 1940s.

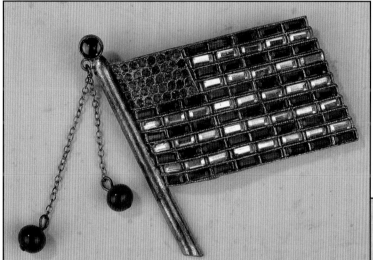

Wonderful American flag pin with red and white baguette stones. 2 red glass balls dangle from chains. WWII period.

3 Silver and gold flag pole pins with swinging American flags. Trifari. Center is replica, c. 1990. Right and left are c. 1942.

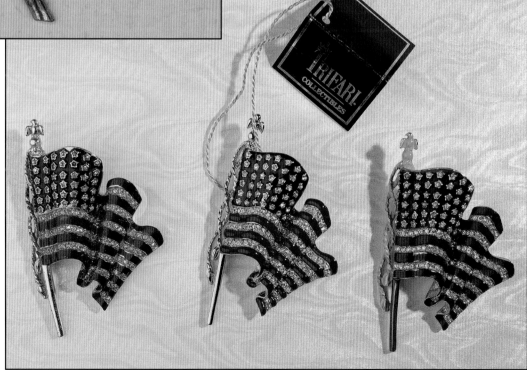

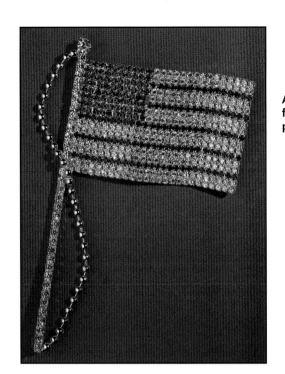

American flag and pole pin.

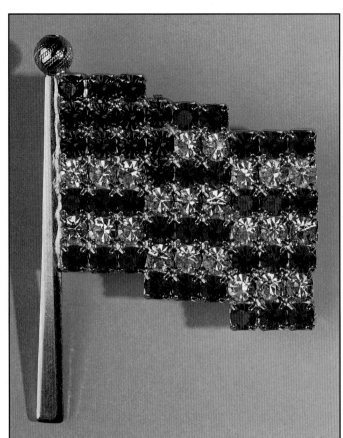

Waving American flag pin. Unsigned.

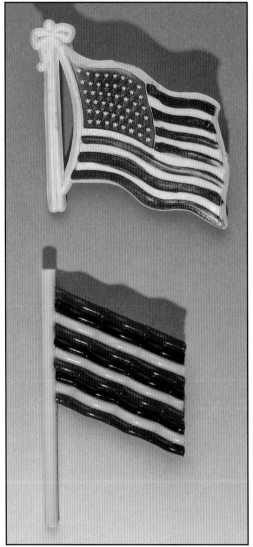

Two American flag pins. Courtesy of Barbara Trujillo.

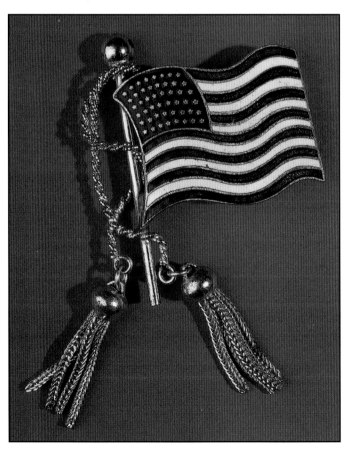

American flag pin with two long tassels. Enamel. 1950s.

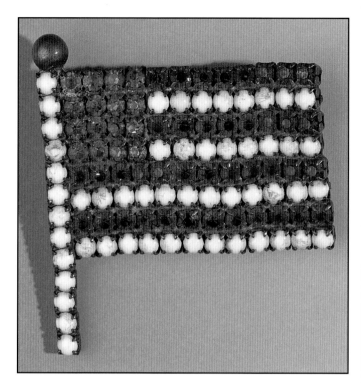
American flag pin. Courtesy of Barbara Trujillo.

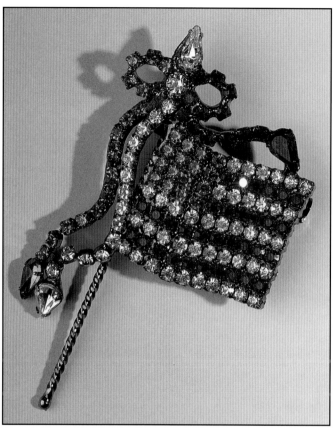
American flag pin with round red, clear, and blue rhinestones. Unsigned. Contemporary.

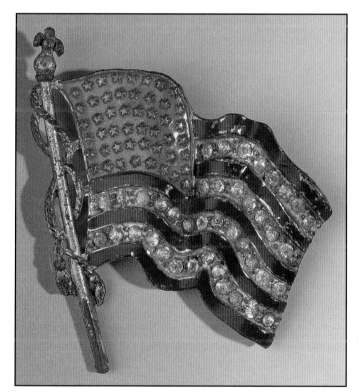
Waving American flag pin. Courtesy of Barbara Trujillo.

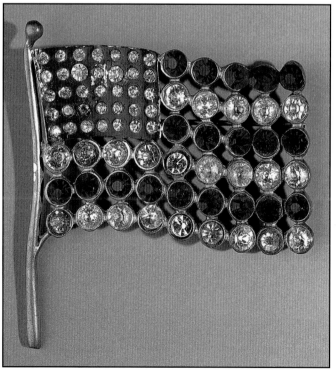
American flag pin. Courtesy of Barbara Trujillo.

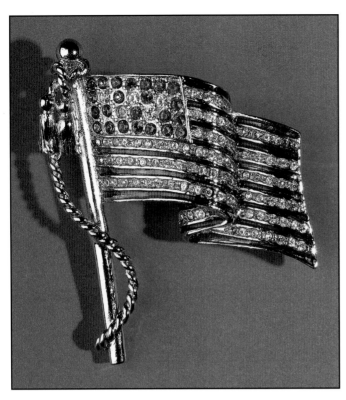

Waving American flag pin. Courtesy of Barbara Trujillo.

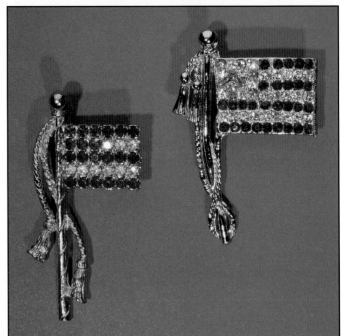

Two gold American flag pins. Unsigned. 1950s-'60s.

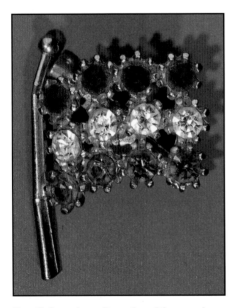

Small American flag pin with round red, clear, and blue rhinestones. Unsigned. 1960s.

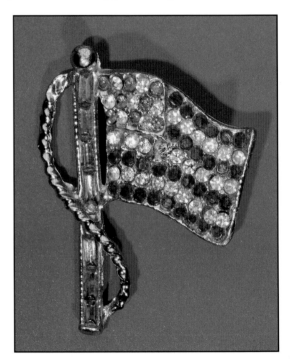

Waving American flag pin with light blue rhinestones in the flag pole. Unsigned. 1960s.

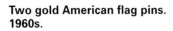

Two gold American flag pins. 1960s.

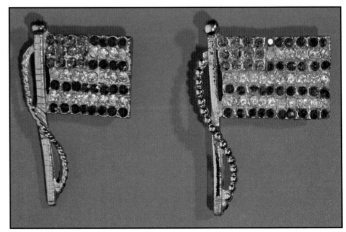

Enameled waving American flag tie
tack. Unsigned. Contemporary.

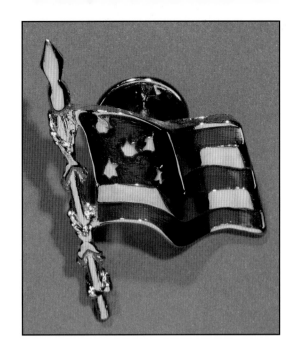

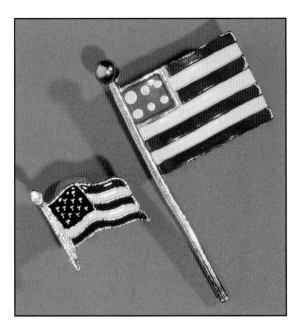

Two American flags. Tiny one is a tie tack, large
one is a pin.

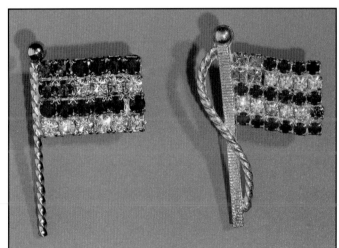

Two gold American flag pins. 1960s.

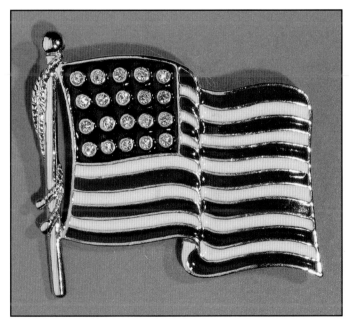

Enameled waving American flag pin. Made in China.
Contemporary.

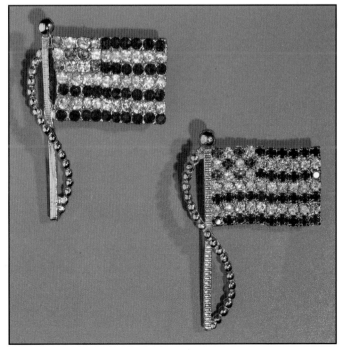

Two American flag pins.
1960s.

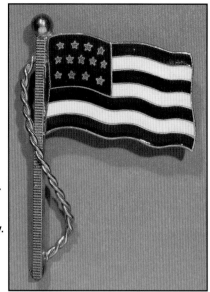

Enameled gold American flag pin in red, white, and blue. Unsigned. Contemporary.

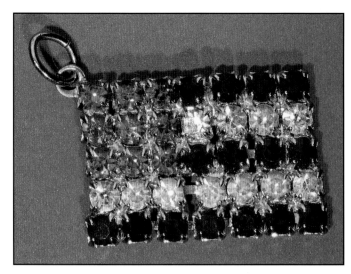

American flag charm. Contemporary.

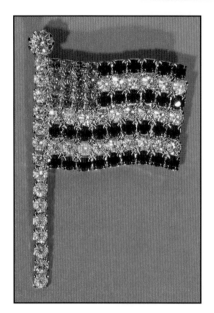

American flag pin. Unsigned. Contemporary.

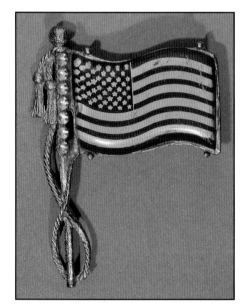

Waving American flag pin. Unsigned. 1960s.

American flag pin with red, clear, and blue rhinestones. 1950s.

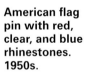

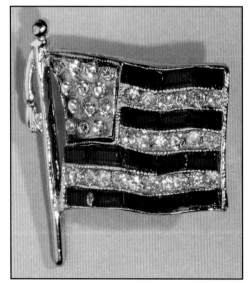

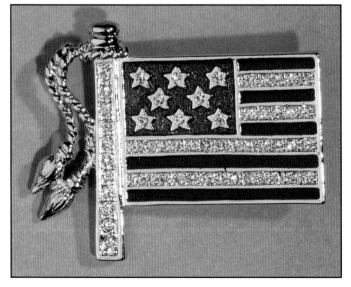

American flag pin. Signed E. Pearl, Thailand. Contemporary.

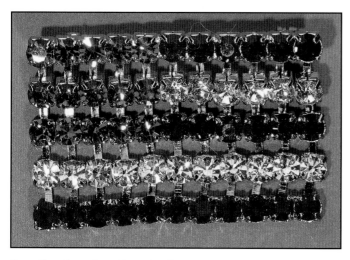

Dangling American flag pin. Contemporary.

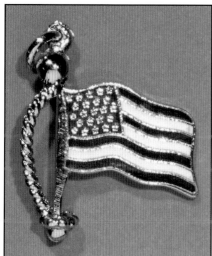

Tiny enameled gold waving American flag charm. Contemporary.

American flag pin with red, clear, and blue rhinestones. Signed Camillot. Contemporary.

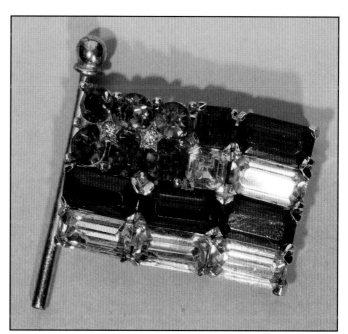

American flag pin. 1940s.

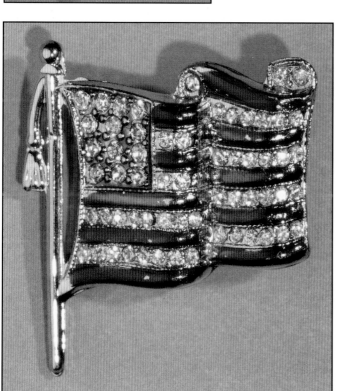

Waving American flag pin. Unsigned. 1940s.

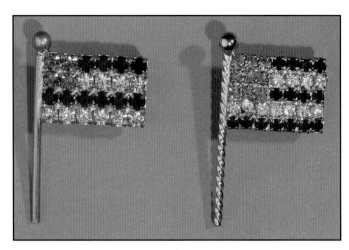

Two American flag pins. 1960s.

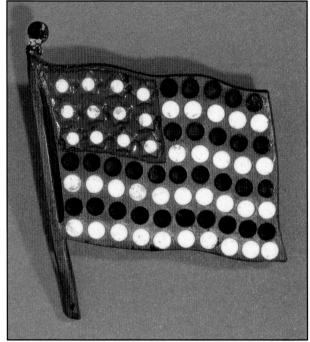

American flag pin in enamel. Unsigned. 1940s.

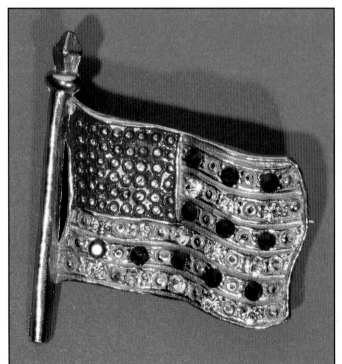

Gold American flag pin.
Unsigned. 1960s.

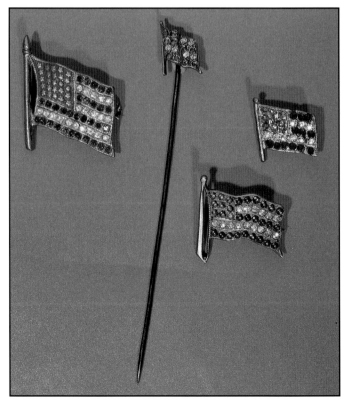

Four American flag pins with
enamel and rhinestones. Tiny stick
pin. Unsigned. 1940s.

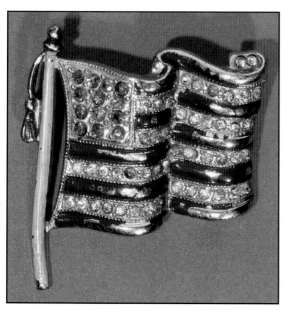

Waving American flag pin. Unsigned. 1940s.

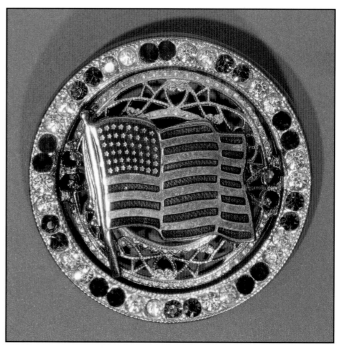

Gold pin with enameled American flag in center and surrounded with red, clear, and blue rhinestones. 1950s.

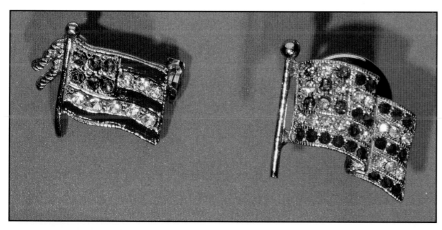

American flag pin with enamel, and tie tack with rhinestones. 1960s.

American flag pin. Unsigned. 1940s.

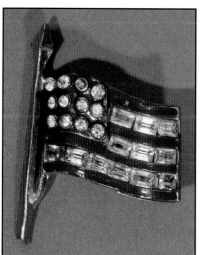

Small enameled American flag pin. Unsigned. 1940s.

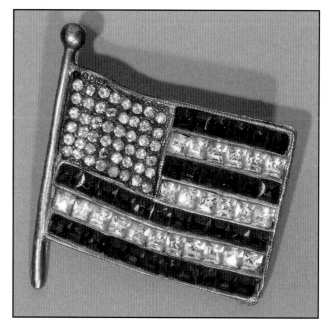

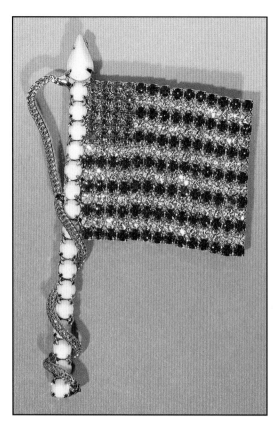

American flag pin with red, clear, and blue rhinestones on white beaded flagpole. Signed by Dominique. Contemporary.

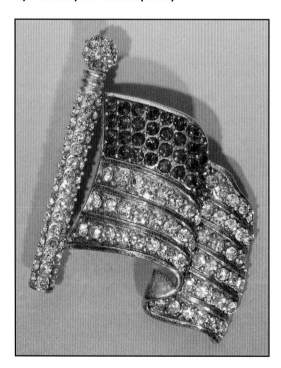

Waving American flag pin. Unsigned. Contemporary.

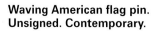
Waving American flag pin. Unsigned. Contemporary.

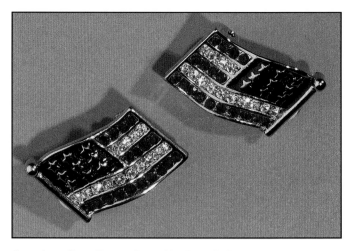

American flag clip earrings. Unsigned. Contemporary.

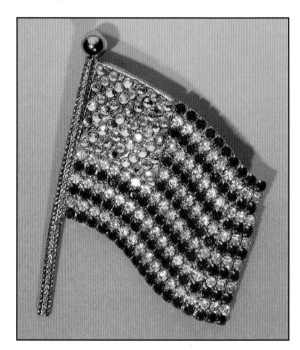

American flag with red, clear, and blue rhinestones. Unsigned. 1960s.

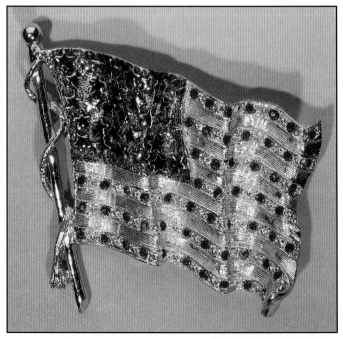

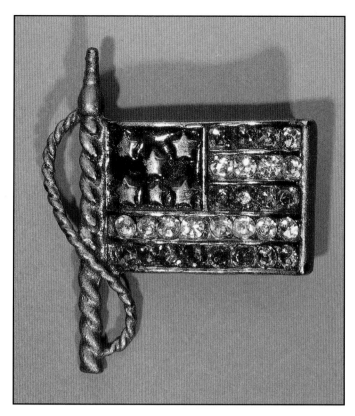

American flag pin in enamel and rhinestones. Unsigned. 1950s.

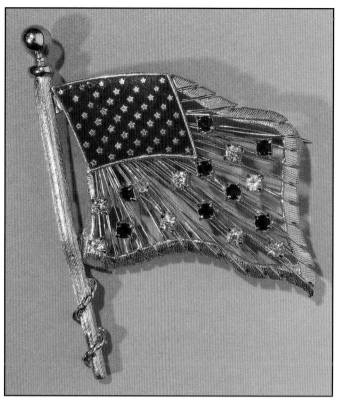

Waving American flag pin. Unsigned. 1960s.

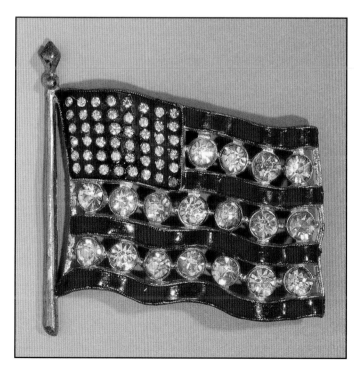

American flag with red and blue enamel and clear rhinestones. Unsigned. 1940s.

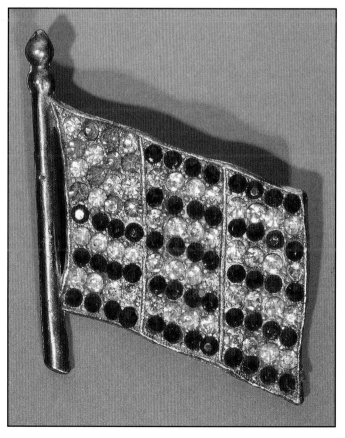

American flag pin. Unmarked. 1940s.

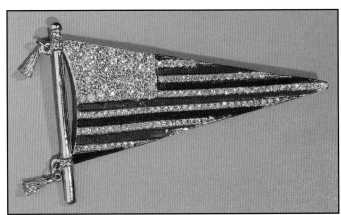

Gold American flag pendant. Signed Polcini.

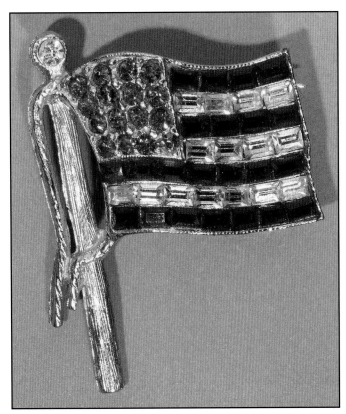

American flag pin. © Pedo.

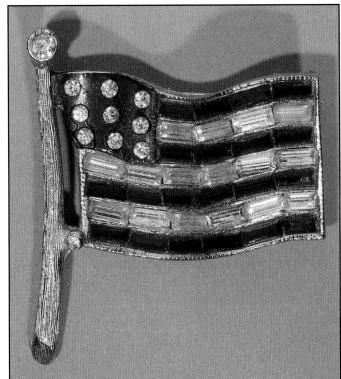

American flag pin with baguette rhinestones and blue enamel.

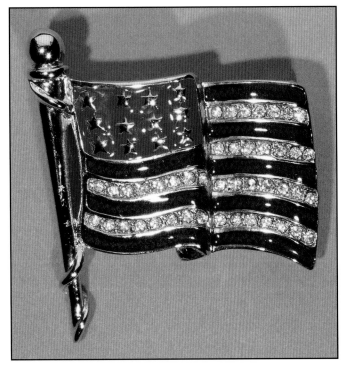

Waving American flag pin. Unsigned. Contemporary.

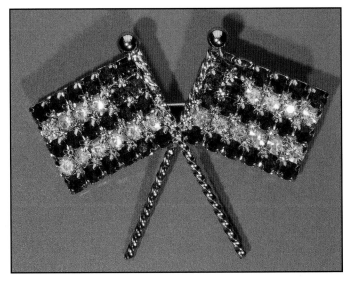

Two American flags crossed at the poles. Marked Hobé c. 1966.

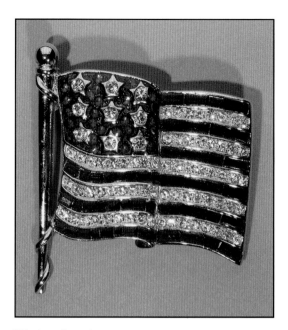

Waving American flag pin. Unsigned. Contemporary.

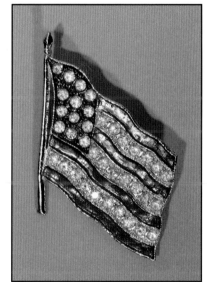

American flag pin with red enamel and clear rhinestones. 1940s.

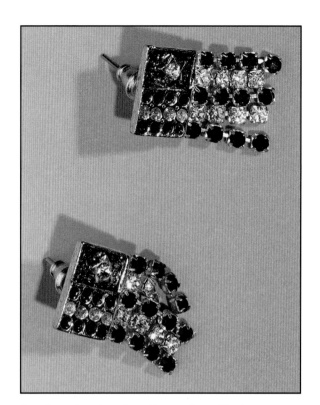

Small waving American flag earrings. Contemporary.

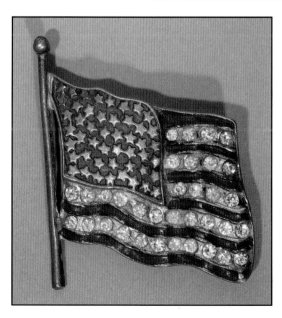

American flag pin. Enamel. Unsigned. 1940.

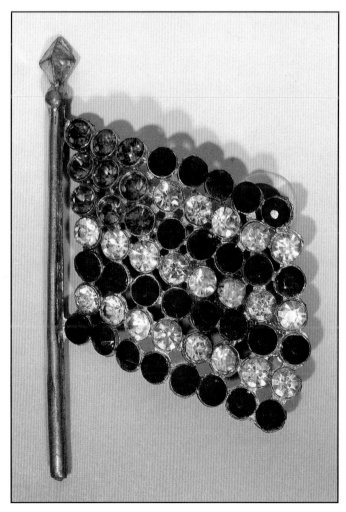

American flag pin with round red, clear, and blue rhinestones. Unsigned. 1940s.

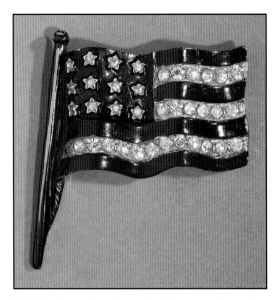

Waving American flag pin with enamels and rhinestone. By Trifari.

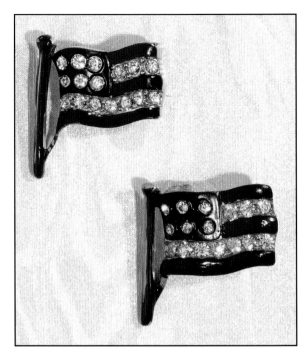

Two small American flag pins in enamel and rhinestones. Both signed Trifari.

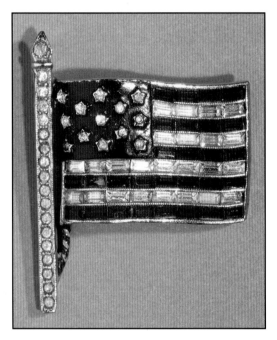

American flag pin with baguettes. Signed Trifari. 1940s.

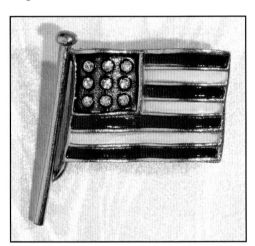

Tiny American flag pin. Signed Trifari.

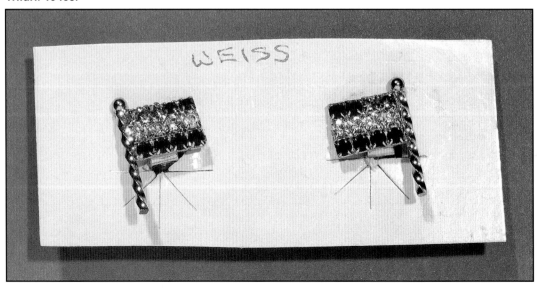

American flag earrings. By Weiss. 1950s.

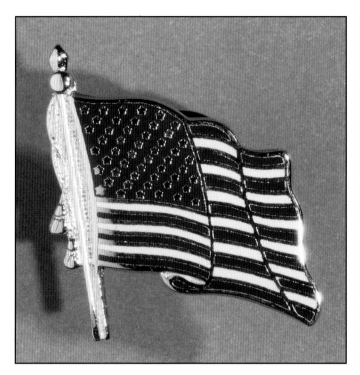

Tiny waving American flag tie tack, all enamel.
Box marked Karatclad.

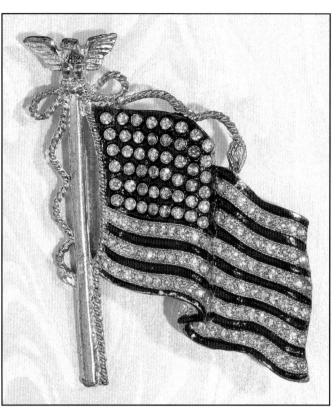

Waving American flag pin with silver eagle sitting atop the
flag pole. Unsigned. 1940s.

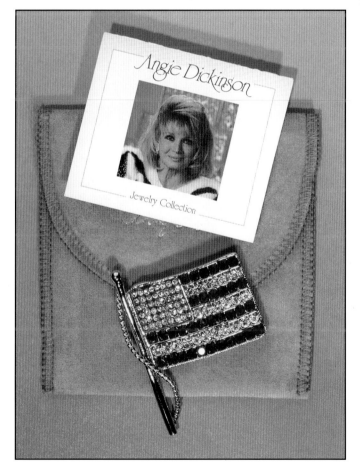

American flag pin from the Angie Dickinson Collection.
Made by Kenneth Jay Lane (sold by QVC), contemporary, in
box.

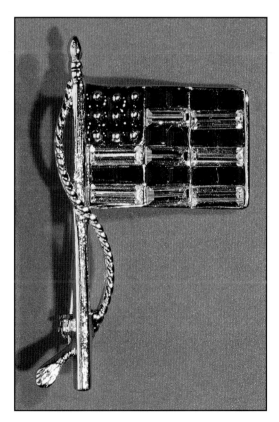

American flag pin. Signed Kirk's Folly.
Made in USA.

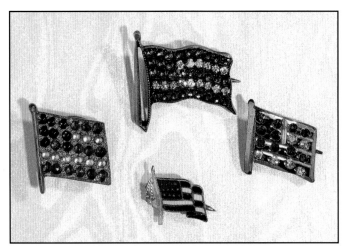

Four small American flag pins. Enamel and rhinestones. 1940s. Top unmarked. Left: lapel stud, marked "Enco." Right: "SHUITE." Bottom: enamel and brass, unmarked.

Bar pin with square-cut rhinestones. Two American flag pins in patriotic colors. Left: sterling, Corocraft. Right: enamel, unsigned. 1940s.

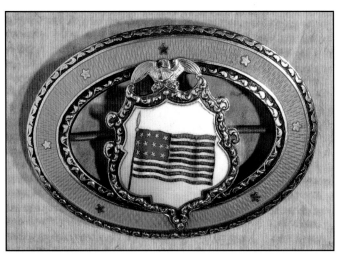

Oval pin with enameled American flag and eagle in enameled turquoise frame, marked Sterling.

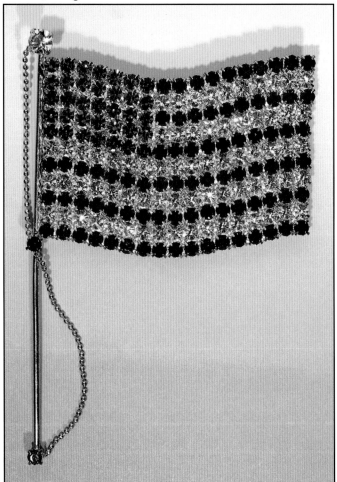

American flag pin with red, clear, and blue rhinestones. Chain on flag pole.

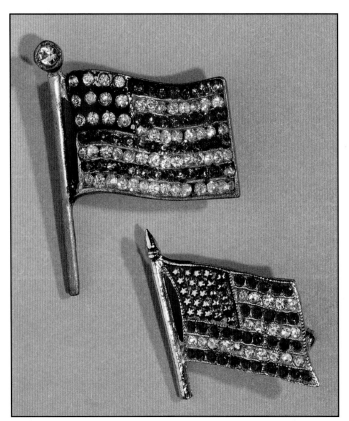

Two small American flag pins with rhinestones.

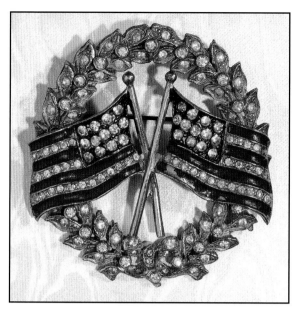

Gold pin with two American flags crossed at the poles in a wreath. Unsigned. 1930.

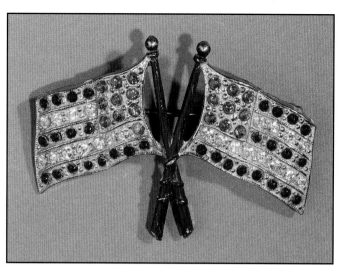

Pin with crisscrossing American flags in metal. 1930s.

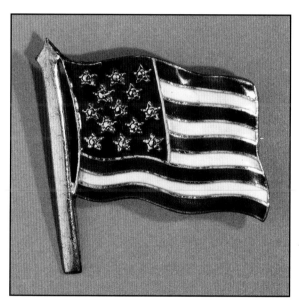

American flag pin.

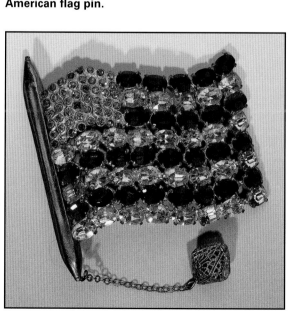
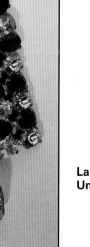

Waving American flag pin with dangling tassels, enameled. 1940s.

Large American flag pin. 2 1-2" w. Unsigned. 1940s.

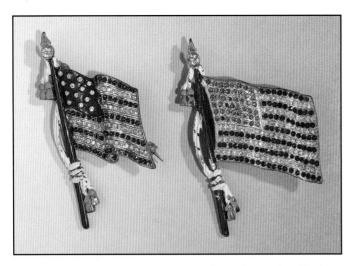

Rippling flag pins with enamel tassels on flag poles. Both unsigned, 1930s.

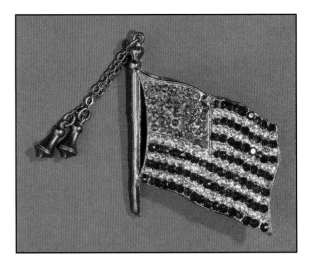

American flag pin with round cut blue, clear, and red rhinestones. Unmarked. 1940s.

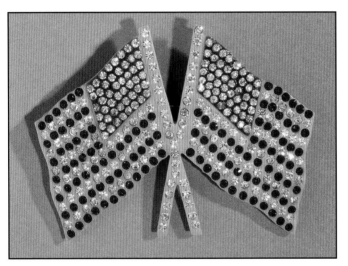

Plastic pin with crossed American flags.

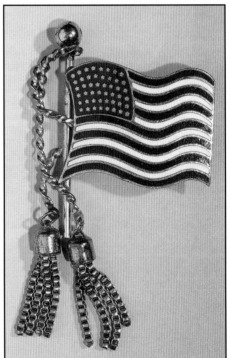

Waving American flag. Enamel. 1950s. Unsigned.

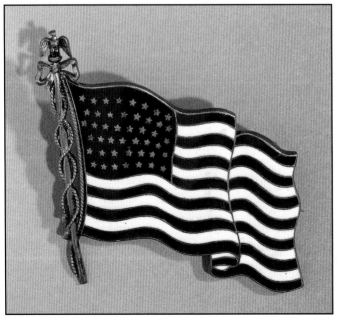

Waving American flag pin. All enamel, sterling, unmarked. 1940s.

American flag pin with round and square cut rhinestones. Unsigned. 1940s.

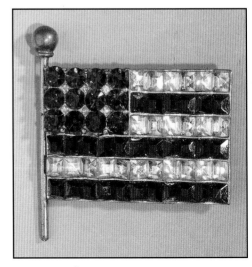

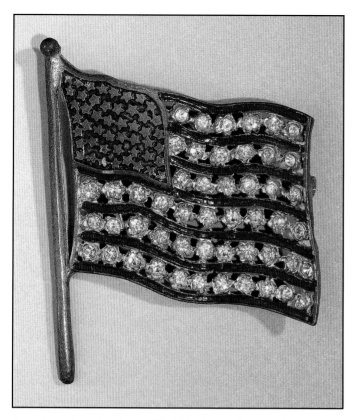

American flag pin. Enamel field and metal stars. Unsigned. 1930s.

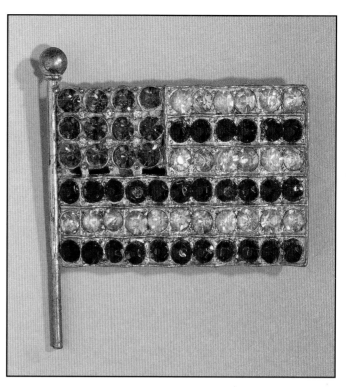

Silver American flag pin with round rhinestones. Unsigned. 1940s.

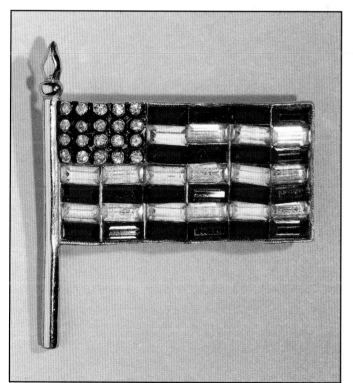

American flag pin. Unsigned. 1940s.

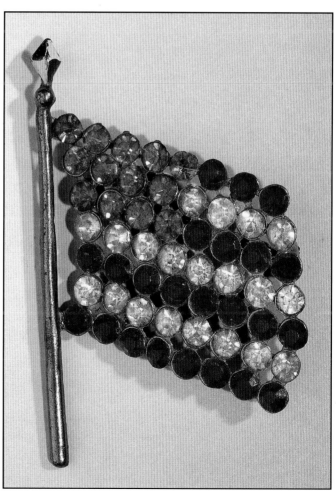

American flag pin with round rhinestones. Unsigned. 1940s.

American flag pin with round and square rhinestones and hinged tassels. Unsigned. 1940s.

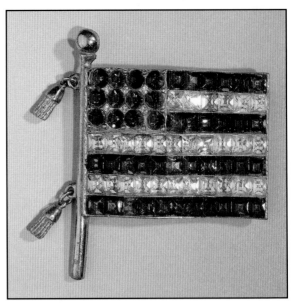

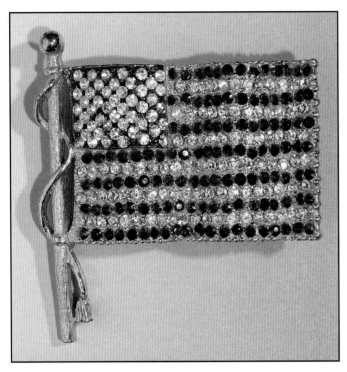

American flag pin with gold flag pole. Enameled blue field,
signed Hattie Carnigie. 1940s.

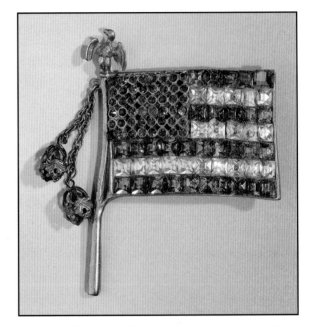

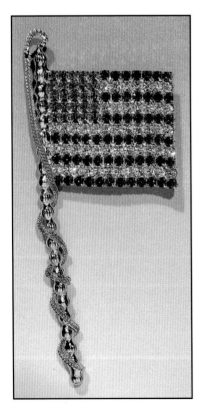

American flag pin
with fancy gold roped
flag pole. Signed
Dominique. 4 1/2" tall.
Contemporary.

American flag pin with round and square cut rhinestones and eagle sitting atop pole; filigree balls.
Unsigned. 1940s.

Swaying American
flag and eagle sitting
atop the pole. Enam-
el and blue dots with
clear rhinestones.

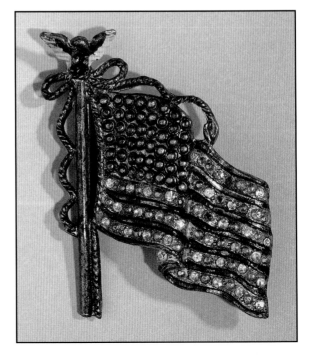

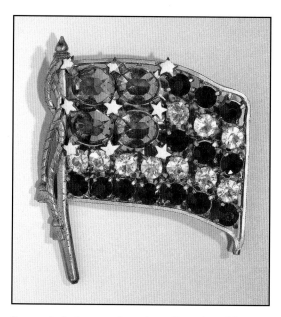

Enameled stars on American flag pin with large round rhinestones. Unsigned. 1940s.

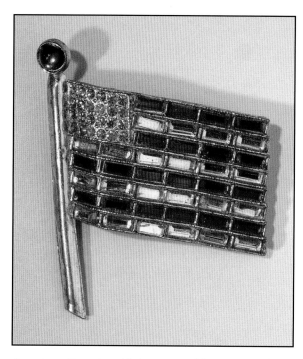

American flag pin with baguette rhinestone stripes. Unsigned, c. 1930.

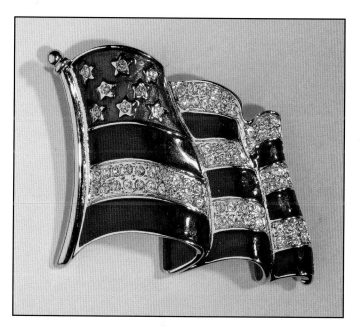

Waving American flag pin. Enamel and rhinestone. Signed by Ann Hand, contemporary.

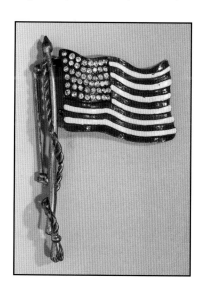

Hinged silver American flag pin. Enamel and rhinestones. c. 1930, unsigned.

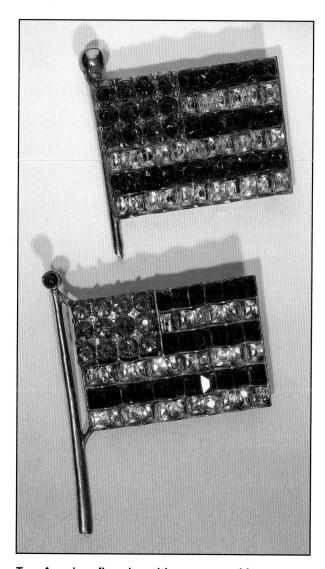

Two American flag pins with square cut rhinestone stripes. Both unsigned, 1940s.

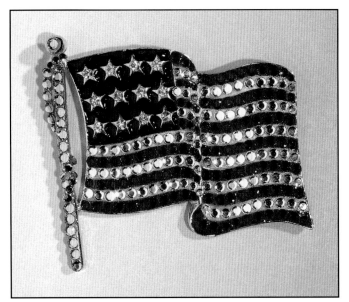

Wonderful contemporary waving American flag pin. Lots of sparkle! Unsigned.

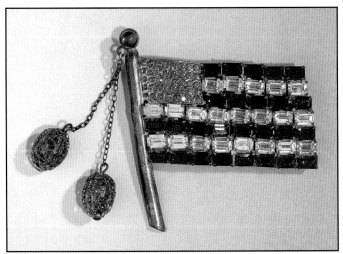

American flag pin with square cut rhinestone stripes, blue enamel field. Unsigned. 1940s.

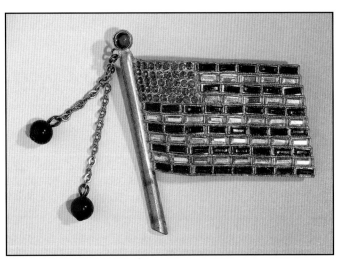

American flag pin with baguette rhinestone stripes. Unsigned. 1940s.

American flag pin with 2 filigree balls. Unsigned. 1940s.

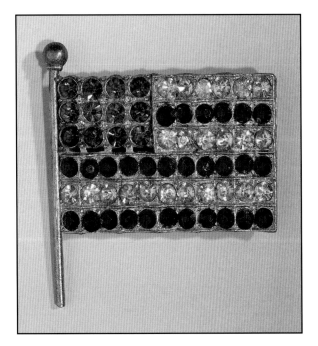

Gold American flag pin with round rhinestones. Unsigned. 1940s.

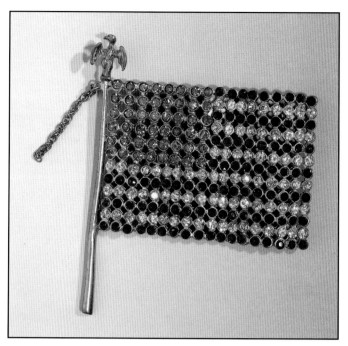

American flag pin with eagle on top of the flag pole. Unsigned. 1940s.

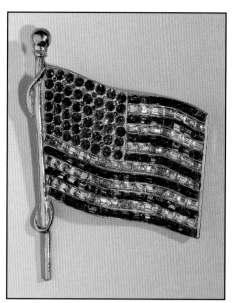

American flag pin. Unsigned. 1940s.

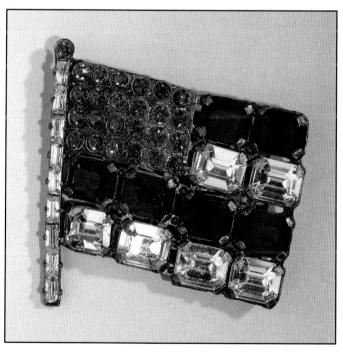

American flag pin with stripes in large cut rhinestones. Unsigned. 1950s.

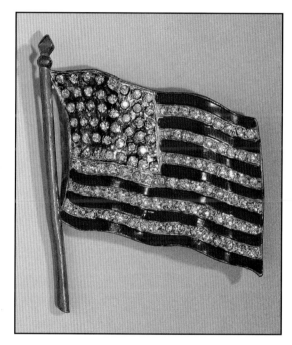

American flag pin. Enamel and rhinestones. Unsigned. 1940s.

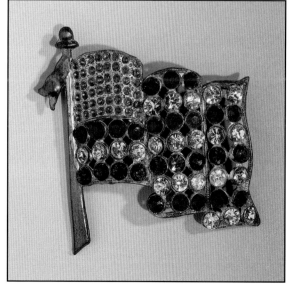

American flag pin with circular cut rhinestones. Unsigned. 1940s.

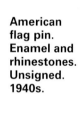
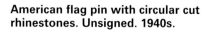

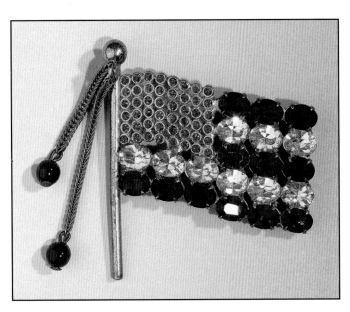

American flag pin with large oval-cut rhinestones for stripes. Unsigned. 1940s.

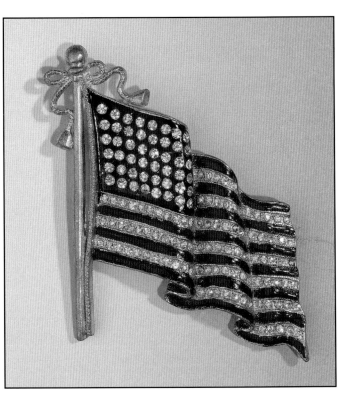

American flag pin in enamel and rhinestone. Unsigned. 1940s.

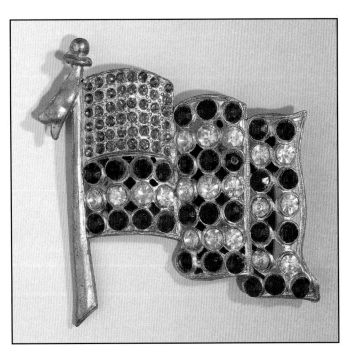

American flag pin with round rhinestones. Unsigned. 1940s.

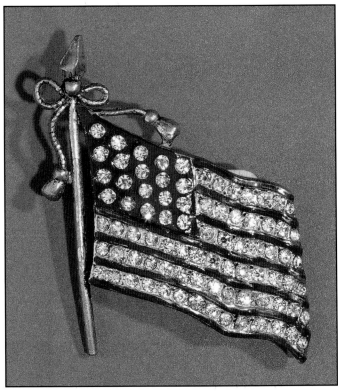

Waving American flag pin. Enamel and rhinestones. Unmarked. 1930s.

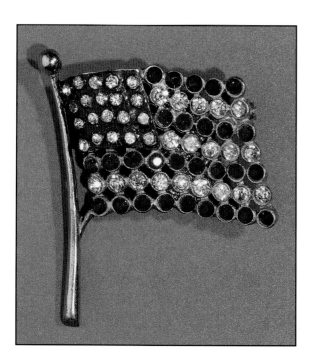

American flag pin with round rhinestones. Marked Calvaire. 1940s.

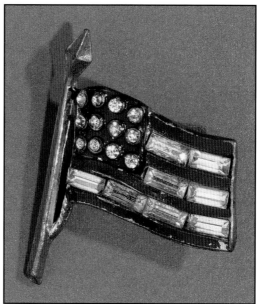

American flag pin. Enamel and baguettes. Unmarked. 1940s.

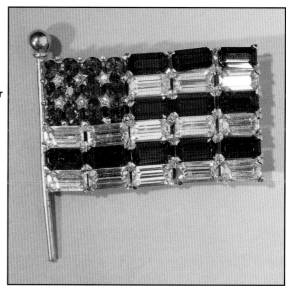

Spectacular American flag pin. 1940s.

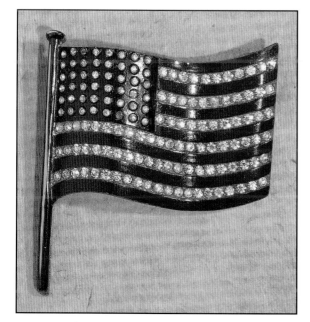

Waving American flag pin in enamel with clear rhinestones. Signed Trifari. 1940s.

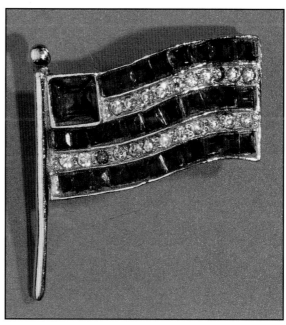

American flag pin with round and square-cut rhinestones. Unmarked. 1940s.

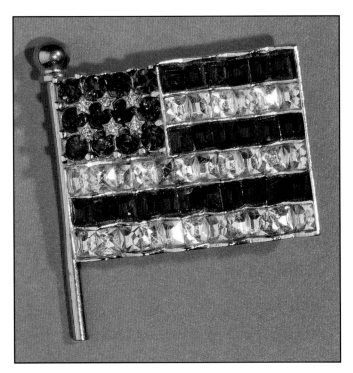

American flag pin with square cut rhinestones.
Unmarked. 1940s.

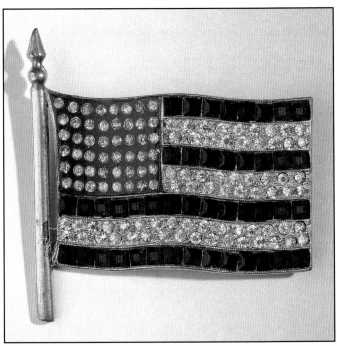

Outstanding American flag and pole pin, 1940s.

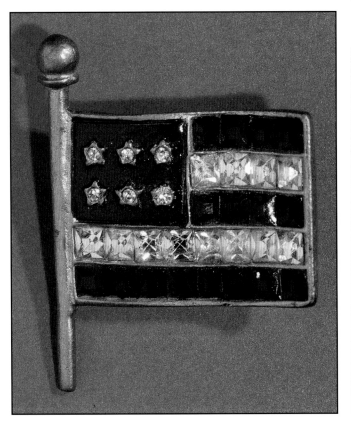

Enamel and rhinestone American flag pin with 6 stars.
Unmarked. 1940s.

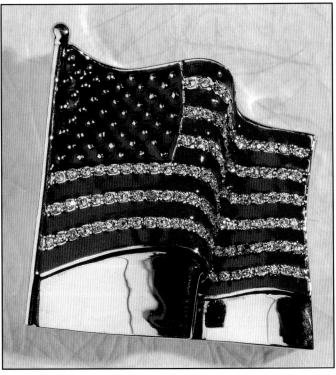

Magnetic box. Contemporary.

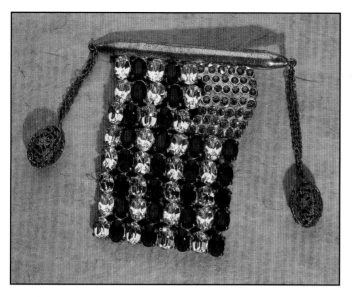

American flag pin. Unsigned.

American flag pin.

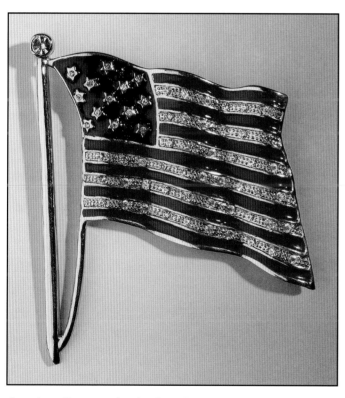

American flag on pole pin. Contemporary.

American flag pin with square cut red, clear, and blue rhinestones. Unsigned. 1940s.

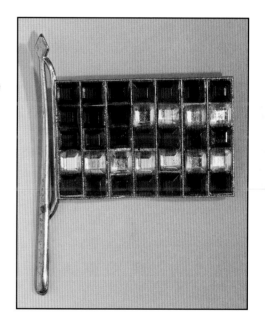

American flag pin. Unsigned. 1940s.

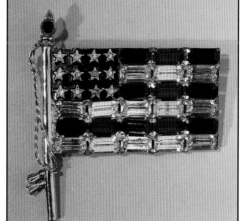

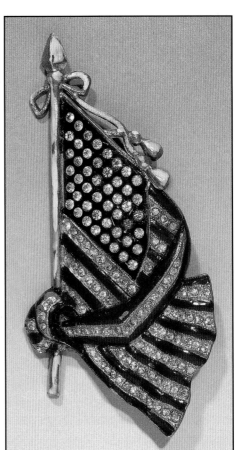

American flag and silver flag pole. 3 1/2" tall. Unsigned. 1940s.

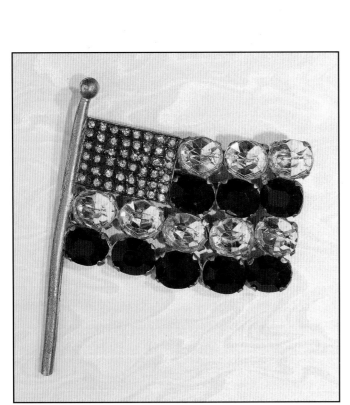

American flag on pole pin. Very large oval stones, unsigned. 1940s.

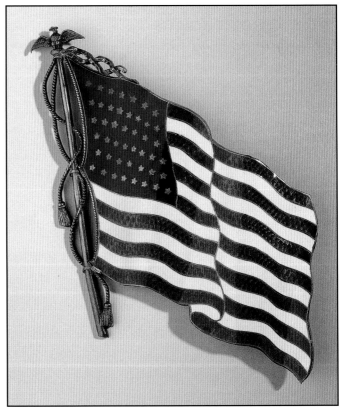

American flag with eagle sitting atop the flag pole pin. Nicely enameled, sterling, marked Hamilton & Diesinger, 3 1/4" x 2 1/2".

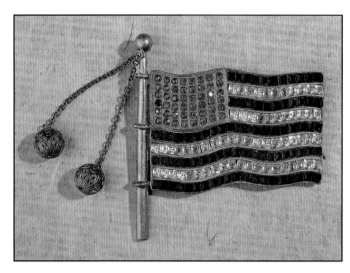

Pole and American flag pin, unsigned. 1940s. Two filigree balls hanging from flag pole.

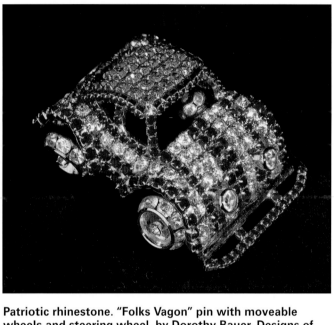

Patriotic rhinestone. "Folks Vagon" pin with moveable wheels and steering wheel, by Dorothy Bauer. Designs of Berkeley, CA. Contemporary.

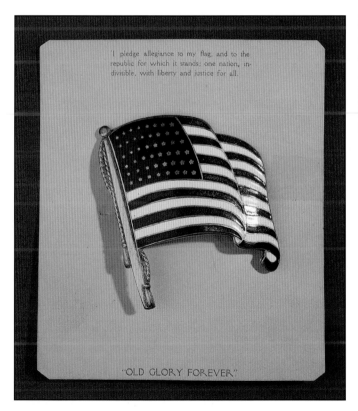

"Old Glory Forever" pin. Enameled, on yellow metal. Unmarked.

Purse pin in American flag theme. Unsigned. Contemporary.

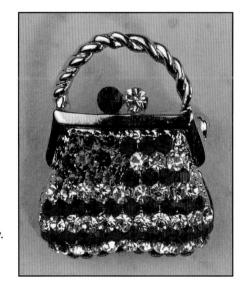

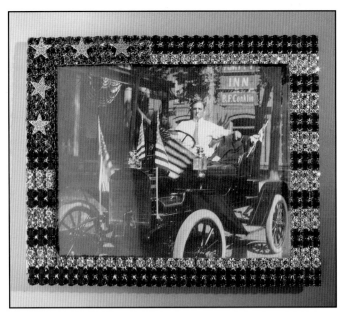

Fabulous photo frame with American flag theme. 7 3/4" x 6 1/4". By CA contemporary designer. Dorothy Bauer. On a personal note, the man in this photo is my paternal grandfather, Frank Lambert Whitson. Does this suggest my love of flags may be a genetic thing?

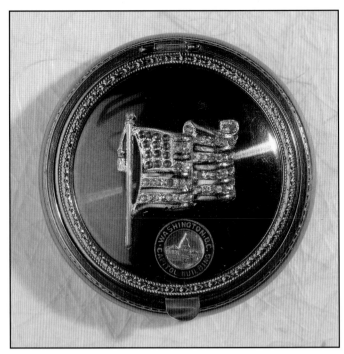

Compact with American flag and Washington, D.C. Capitol building. World War II period.

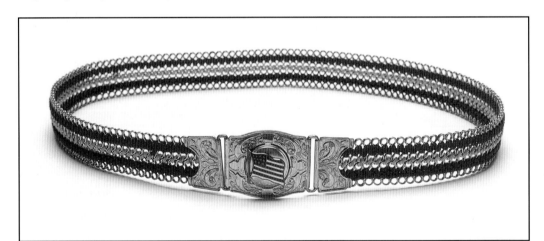

Gold wire and red, white, and blue cord expansion belt with a gold buckle supporting an enameled flag. 1940s.

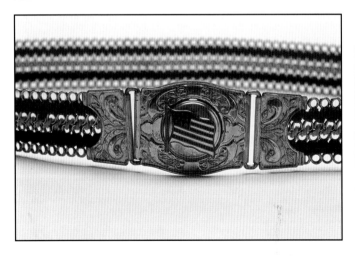

Gold compact with American flag swinging on pole. World War II period.

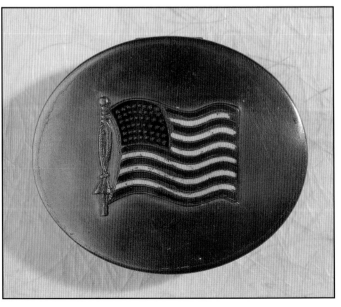

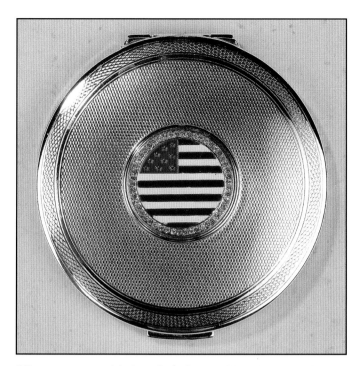

Silver compact with American flag emblem in center. By Stratton. Contemporary.

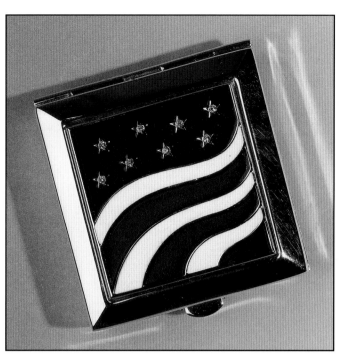

American flag compact from Estee Lauder. "America the Beautiful". 2002.

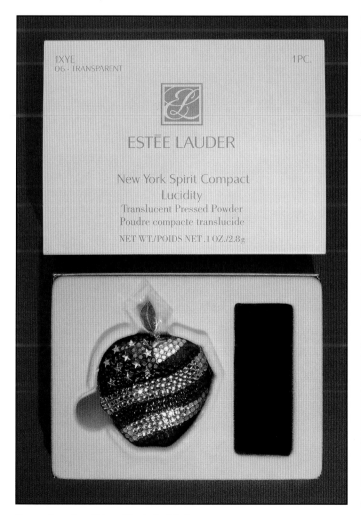

Estee Lauder "New York Spirit" compact.

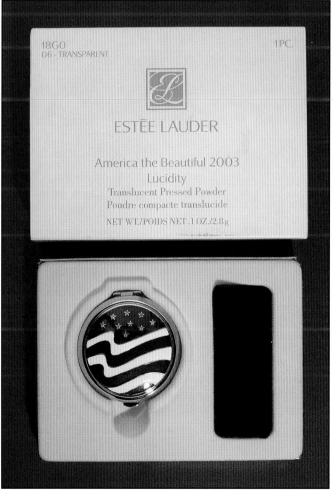

Estee Lauder "America the Beautiful" 2003 Lucidity compact.

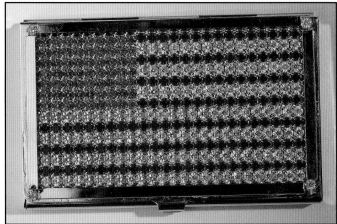

American flag card case. 3 3-4" x 2 1-4". Contemporary.

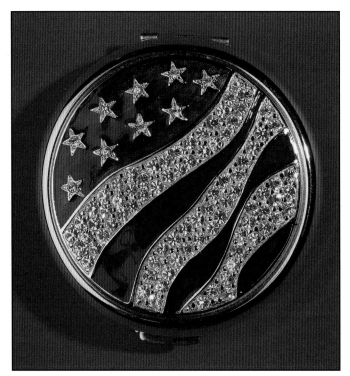

American flag compact by Estee Lauder. Also named "America the Beautiful". Late 1990s.

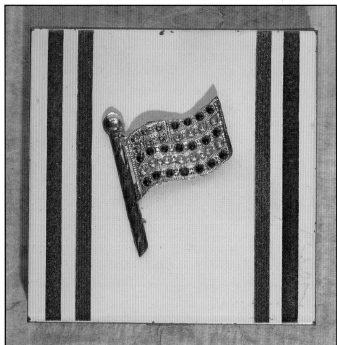

Compact with American flag on pole. World War II period.

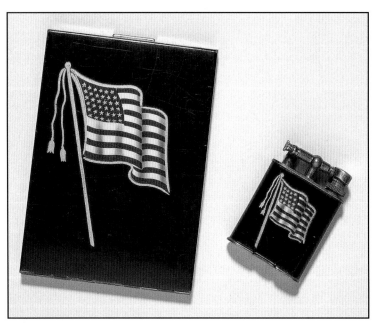

Enameled cigarette case and lighter with an Amercan waving flag decoration. Case unmarked. Lighter marked "The Golden Wheel Lighter US Patents 637855, 666809, other pats pend." 1930s.

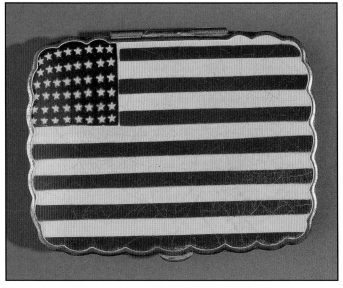

American flag compact. 1940s.

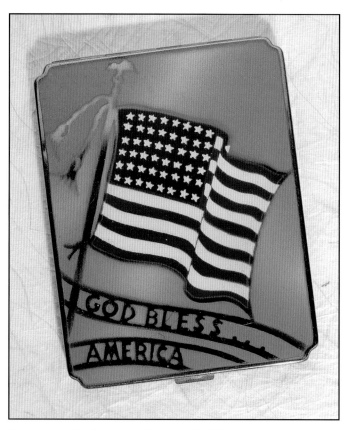

Compact with American flag and God Bless America.
c. 1940s.

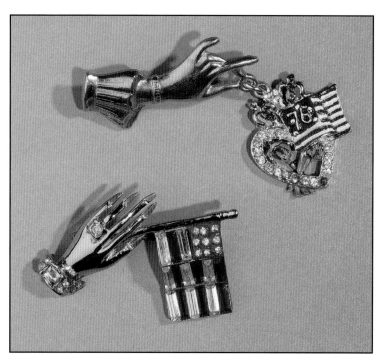

Two pins of woman's hand holding an emblem with a heart and American flag. Top: unsigned, "1976" Bicentennial. Bottom: sterling by Corocraft.

American flag cuff
links. 1960s.

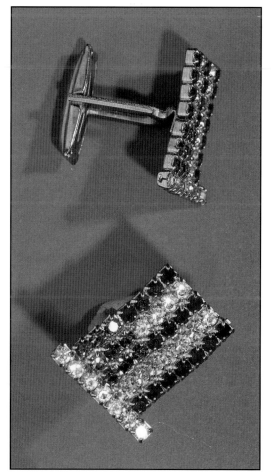

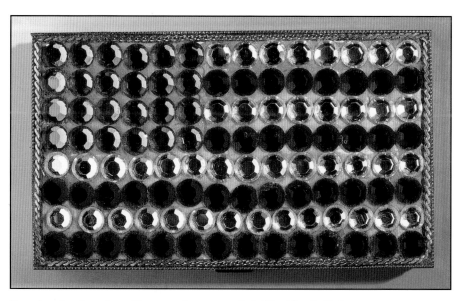

Spectacular American flag evening purse. 5 1-4" x 3" x 3-4" deep.

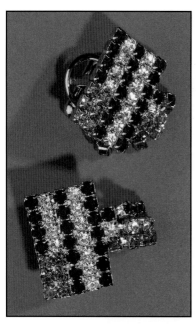

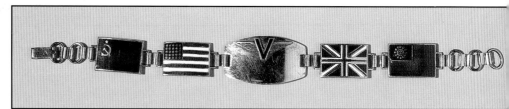

Silver link bracelet with enameled flags of the four W.W.II allies: Russia, USA, Britain, and China. Each link marked "Sterling." Early 1940s.

American flag cuff links with red, clear, and blue rhinestones.

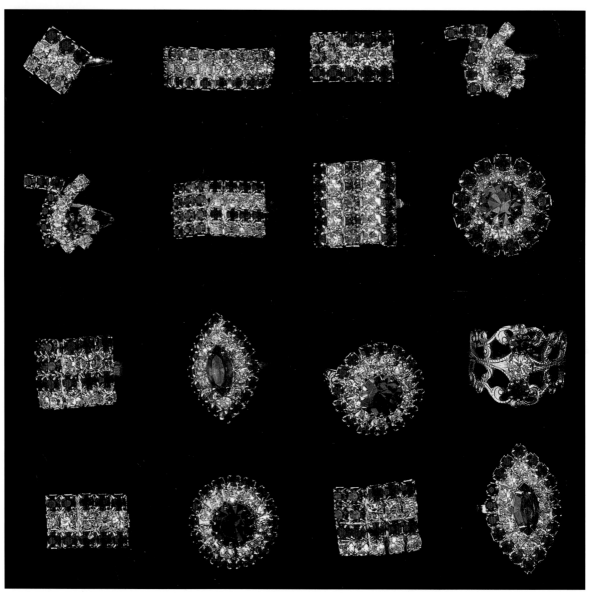

An assortment of rings in patriotic themes, ranging in dates from 1950-1976.

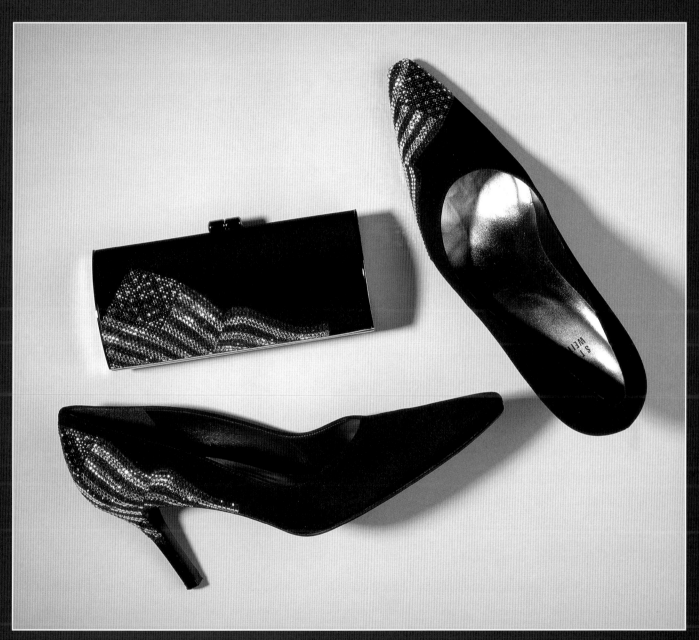

Woman's black silk shoes and matching purse, especially made for author Sandra Whitson. Red, clear, and blue, hand-set, Austrian, flat-backed rhinestones in a waving American flag design are placed on one shoe's toe, the other shoe's heel, and the purse. Designed by Stuart Weitzman for his Pavé Collection. Contemporary.

Silver necklace with American flag. Black plastic plaque, reverse has red, blue, and gold rhinestones.

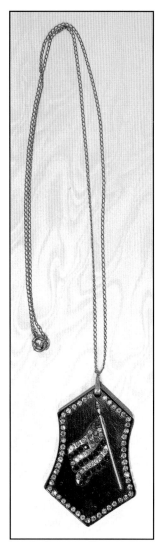

Pin with enameled ribbon and American flag emblem. Sterling. 1940s.

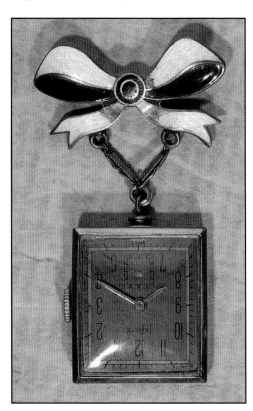

Necklace with American flag theme emblem, like a Fabergé egg, unmarked, contemporary.

Reverse of the pin above, with ribbon and watch face. Sterling. 1940s.

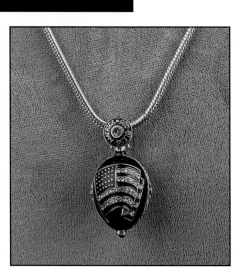

Gold necklace with American flag theme emblem, marked. "God Bless America".

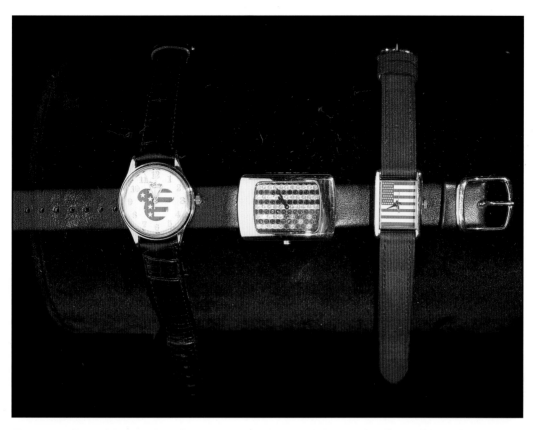

Three watches with American flag themes on the watch face. Left, Mickey Mouse from Disney, contemporary. Center by Fossil, contemporary. Right, unmarked, contemporary.

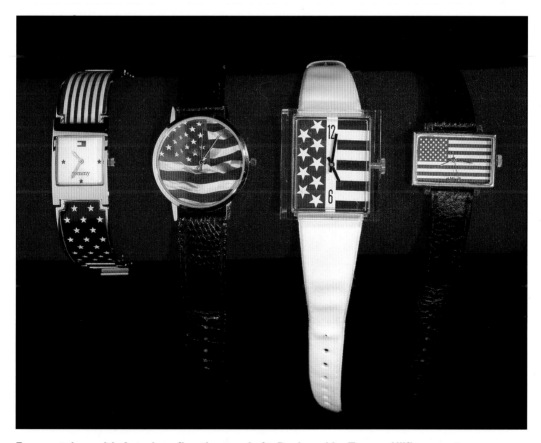

Four watches with American flag themes. Left: Designed by Tommy Hilfiger, contemporary; Black band, contemporary; White band, unmarked, 1960s; "Flag Time" with black band.

Foreign Flags

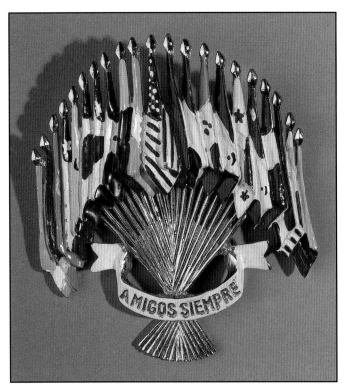

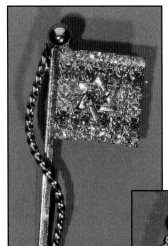

Israeli flag pin with blue and clear rhinestones with a star of David in the center of the flag. Contemporary.

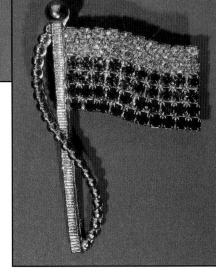

Flags of many nations that reads "Amigos Siempre". League of Nations or United Nations. Signed Coro.

Flag pin with vertical yellow, blue, and red rhinestones. Unsigned. 1960s-70s.

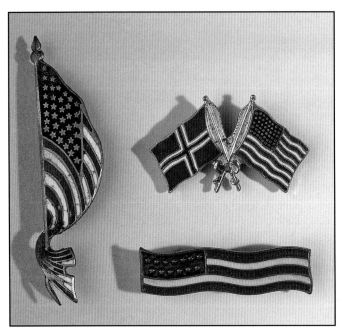

American flag pin. American and British flag pin. American flag pin. Courtesy of Barbara Trujillo.

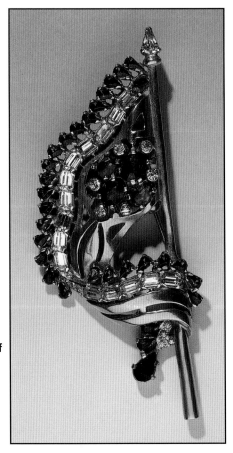

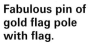

Fabulous pin of gold flag pole with flag.

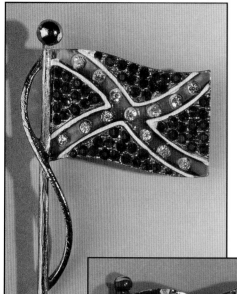

British flag. Courtesy of Barbara Trujillo.

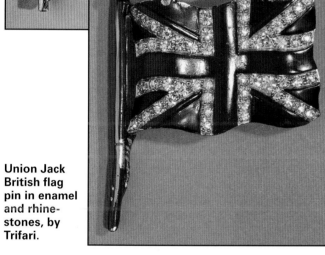

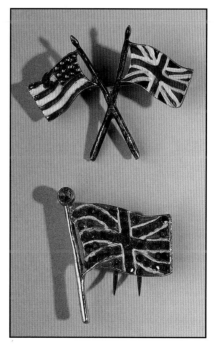

Two tiny gold flag pins. One with crossing x, other stylized American flag. 1970s.

Union Jack British flag pin in enamel and rhinestones, by Trifari.

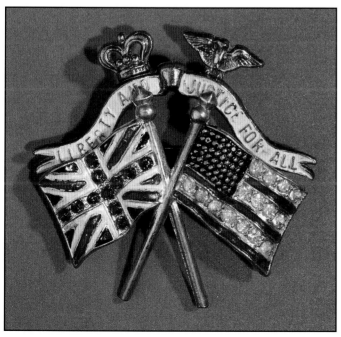

American and British flags crossed at the poles. British flag. Courtesy of Barbara Trujillo.

The British flag with crown atop the flag pole. Crossing American flag with banner saying "Liberty and Justice for All." Unsigned. 1940s.

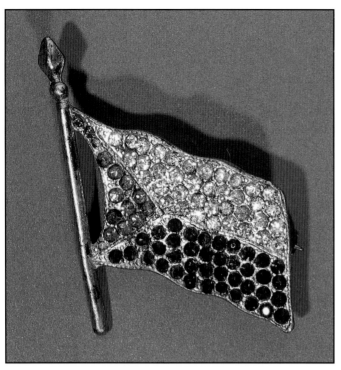

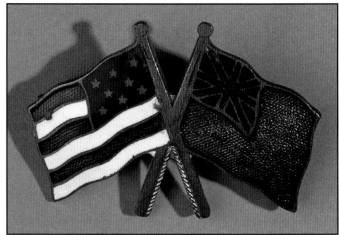

Crossing American flag and British flag pin. 1940s.

Tri-color flag of the Czech Republic as a pin with rhinestones. Contemporary.

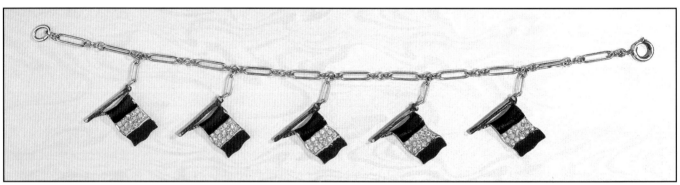

Bracelet with dangling French flag charms with vertical stripes in red, white, and blue. 1940s.

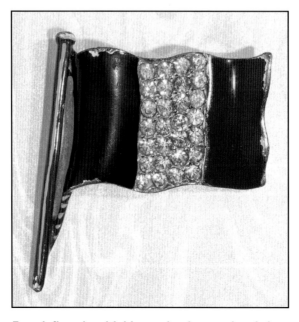

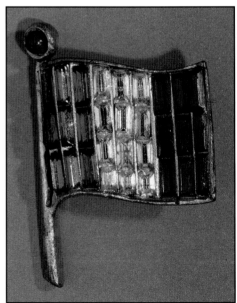

French flag pin with blue and red enamel and clear rhinestone vertical stripes.

French flag pin with 3 vertical rhinestone stripes. Unmarked. 1940s.

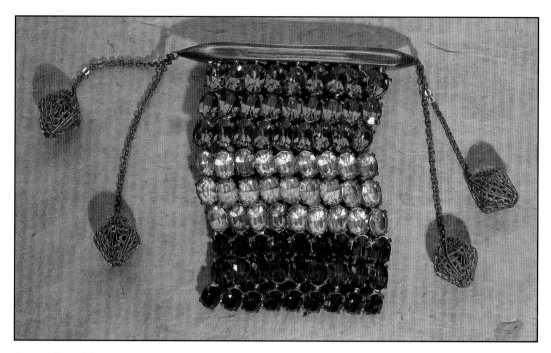

Dress clip with red, white, and blue horizontal stripes. Unsigned. 1940s.

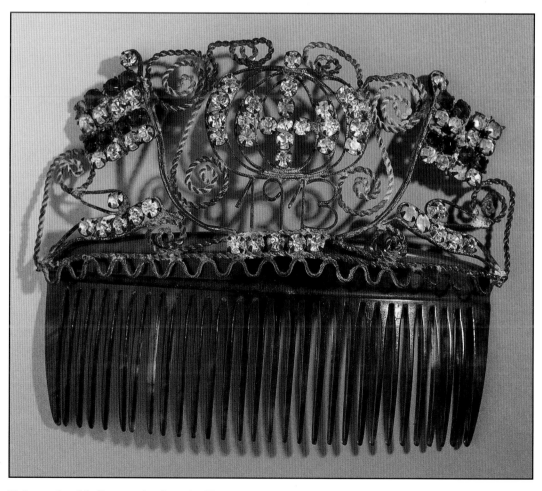

Hair comb with flags on both ends. The year 1913 is part of the comb.

Shields

The patriotic shield is a focal point in the Great Seal of the United States. Its vertical stripes symbolize the original thirteen colonies standing as one. They support and at the same time are joined by the chief, or blue field, at the top of the shield. The blue field represents the President and Congress, the unifying authority under the Articles of Confederation. To the people of the United States, the shield represents patriotism and the strength of American democracy.

Pin in the shape of a shield in enamel with rhinestones. Signed Polcini.

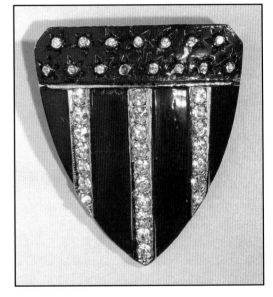

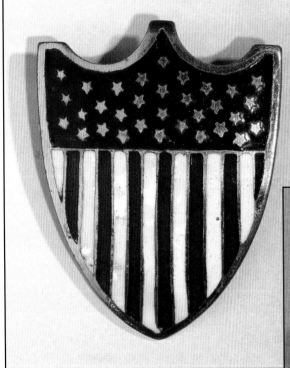

Shield pin with red and white stripes on the bottom and stars on top. All enamel. 1940s.

Rhinestone pin with a shield and olive branches on either side. Unmarked. 1940s.

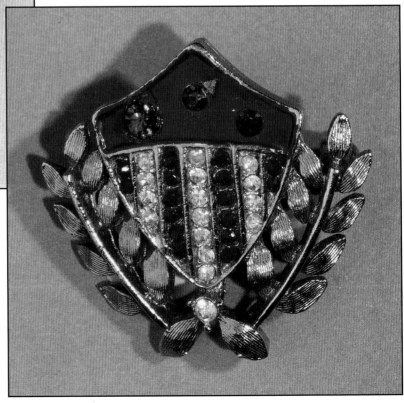

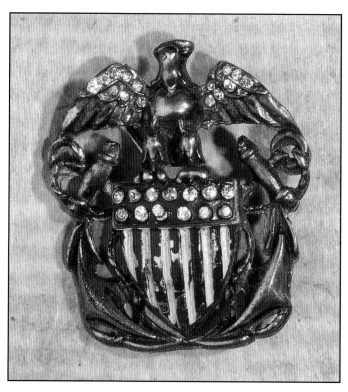

Gold eagle sitting on top of American shield. Signed Sterling and Trifari.

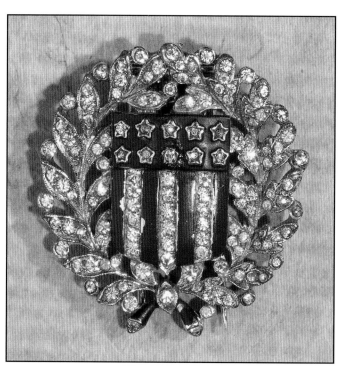

Silver and rhinestone dress clip with flag shield in center and wreath border. Marked Sterling. Trifari.

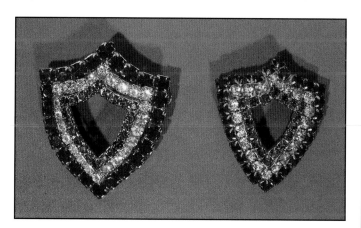

Two pins in the shape of a shield. Unsigned. 1960s.

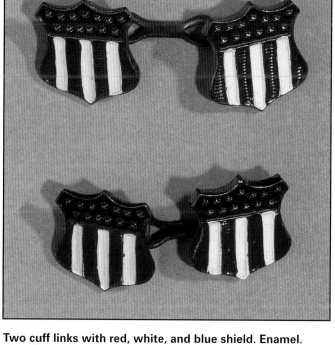

Two cuff links with red, white, and blue shield. Enamel. 1940s.

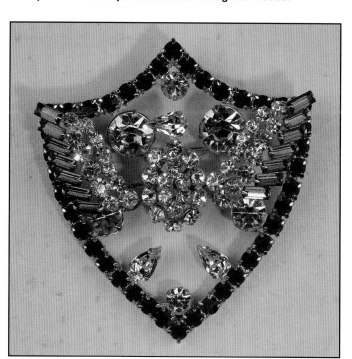

Large pin in the shape of a shield with eagle in the center. Moveable wings. 2 1-2" x 3". Unsigned.

Stars

The national anthem of the United States of America is The Star-Spangled Banner. The flag is sometimes called "the stars and stripes." So, of course, stars that represent the states are an integral part of patriotic jewelry: pins, earrings, brace- lets, etc. Whereas stars are incorporated on older jewelry; most of the single-star pins are more contemporary. The vintage American costume jewelry manufacturing company Trifari made a wonderful star pin, which is pictured on page 58.

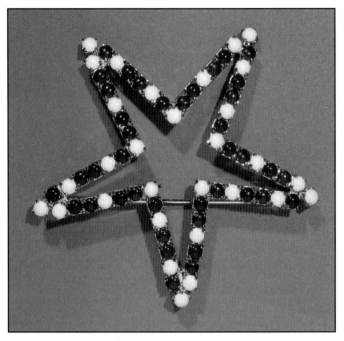

Star pin with red, white milk glass, and blue beads. Contemporary.

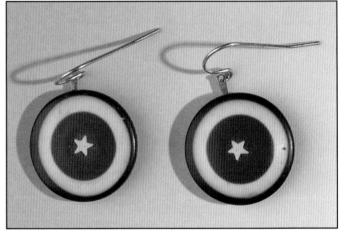

Earrings with a star in the center. Courtesy of Barbara Trujillo.

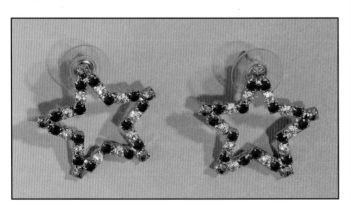

Star shaped earrings by Dorothy Bauer.

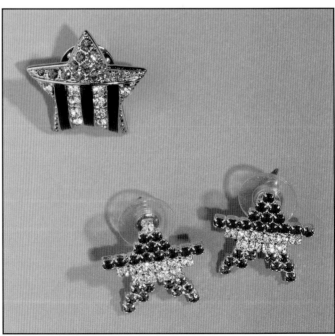

Lapel pin in the shape of a star and pair of earrings. Unsigned. Contemporary.

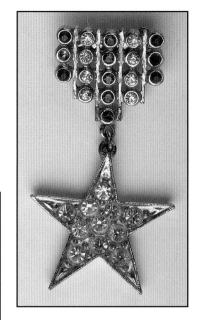

Silver metal military decoration of a red, white, and blue striped rhinestone ribbon design and a pendant star in clear rhinestones. 1940s.

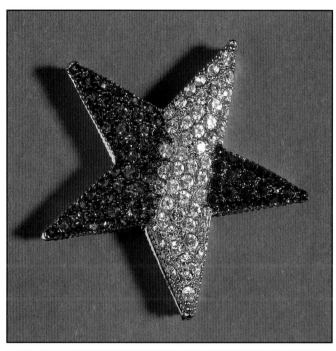

2-part, star-shaped gold metal box with pavé rhinestones on the top, magnetic closure. 3" wide. Contemporary.

Lite Brights star-shaped button covers. Contemporary.

Celluloid pin with three stars, blue and red paint. Unmarked. 1940s.

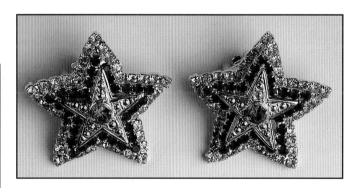

Star earrings of gold metal with three layers of white, red, and blue rhinestones. 1950s.

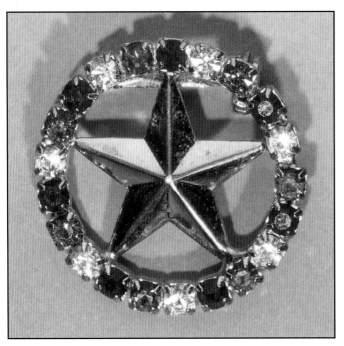

Round pin with gold star in center surrounded by red, clear, and blue rhinestones. Unmarked. 1960s.

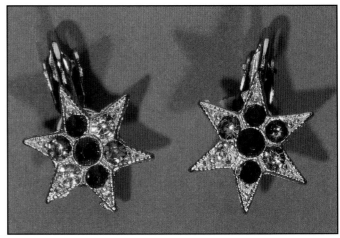

Star-shaped earrings with red, clear, and blue rhinestones. 1950s.

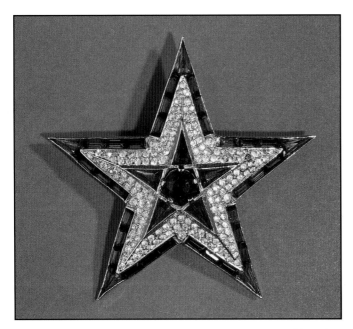

Rare star pin with red, clear, and blue rhinestones. Signed Trifari.

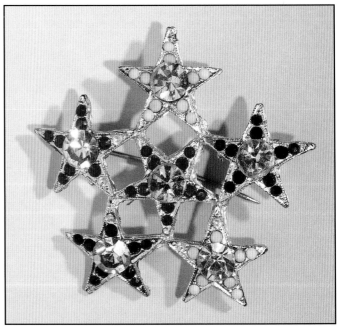

Connecting silver stars with patriotic colored rhinestones. Unsigned. Contemporary.

Ribbons

Ribbons, banners, and scrolls with red, white, and blue fields and stars and stripes are unfurled during patriotic celebrations. They appear on all kinds of American decorations. Accordingly, American patriotic pins often incorporate ribbons, banners, and scrolls to voice deeply felt sentiments. They can add drama and excitement to otherwise ordinary pieces.

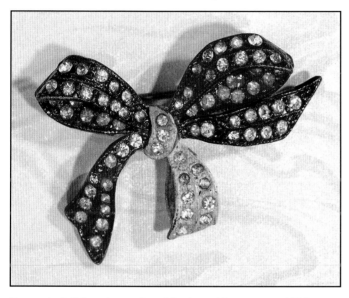

Enameled ribbon bow pin with clear rhinestones. 1930s.

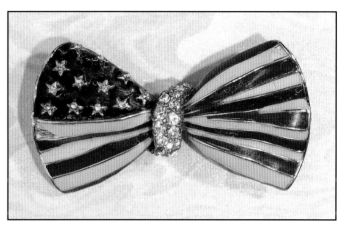

Bow pin with American flag, enamel and rhinestone. Marked Ciner. 1960s.

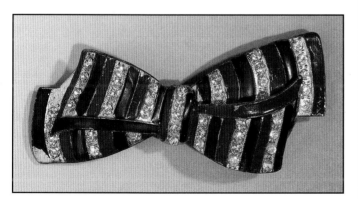

Bow pin with red, clear, and blue stripes. Enamel. Unmarked. 1940s.

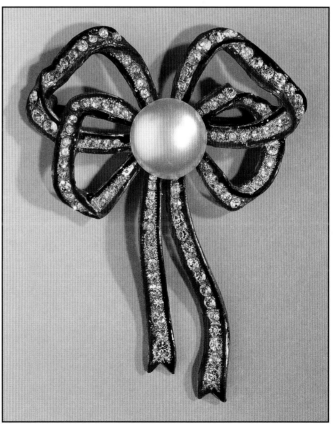

Bow pin in red, white, and blue with pearl center. Unmarked. 1940s.

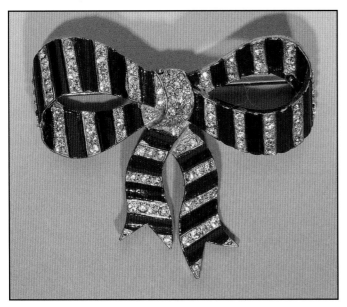

Bow pin in red, white, and blue enamel and rhinestones. Unmarked. 1940s.

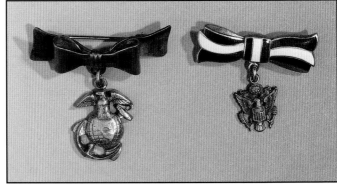

Two metal bow pins with attached eagle emblem pendants. Marine insignia. Army insignia. Sterling.

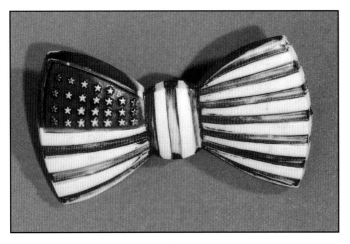

Plastic bow pin in American flag theme. 1950s.

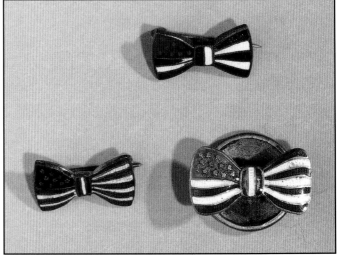

Three bow pins. One an enameled lapel stud, two are tiny straight pins, unmarked. 1940s.

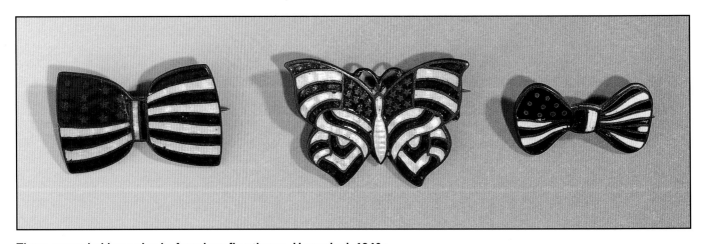

Three enameled bow pins in American flag theme. Unmarked. 1940s.

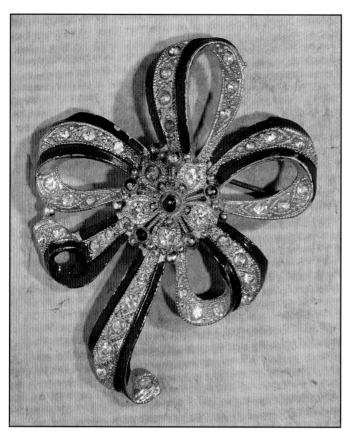

Bow pin in patriotic colors. Unmarked. 1940s.

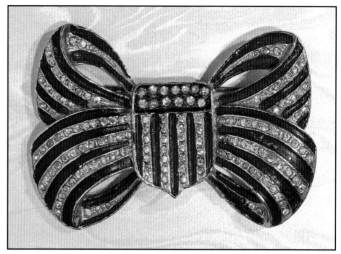

Bow pin with American flag theme shield.

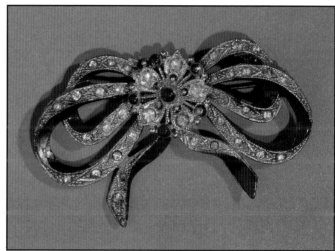

Ribbon bow pin with enamel. Unsigned. 1940s.

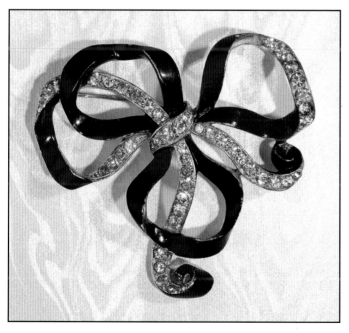

Ribbon bow pin in red, clear, and blue. By Trifari.

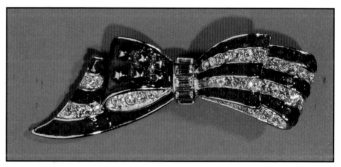

Pin of American flag in the shape of a bow. Unsigned. Contemporary.

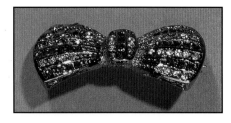

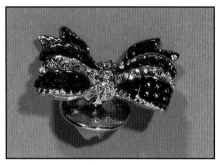

Two small pins in the shape of a bow. Top: gold, unsigned, contemporary. Bottom: B & W, Butler & Wilson, 1970s.

Compact that resembles a pocket watch with a bow on the cover in red, white, and blue rhinestones. 1950s.

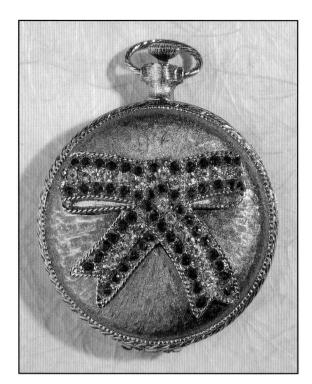

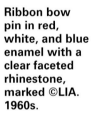

Ribbon bow pin in red, white, and blue enamel with a clear faceted rhinestone, marked ©LIA. 1960s.

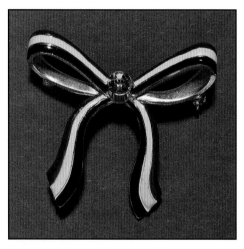

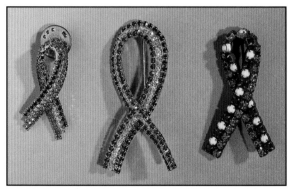

Patriotic looped ribbons with red, white, and blue stones. One lapel pin and two straight pins. 2 unsigned. Right one by Dorothy Bauer.

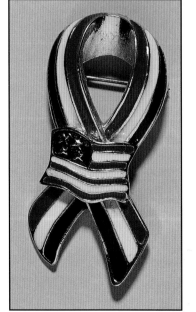

Remember pin of enameled crossing ribbon design and an American flag, marked "KC©." 1970s.

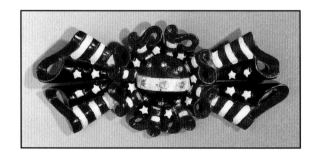

Pin of rolled American flags. Unsigned. c. 1930.

Bow pin in red, white, and blue with clear rhinestones. WWII period.

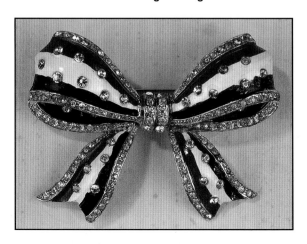

Eagles

The bald eagle is the only eagle unique to North America and was chosen as the National Bird of the United States in 1782. Today, the bald eagle represents its traits of courage, independence, and strength throughout the country.

On July 4, 1776, American patriots Benjamin Franklin, John Adams, and Thomas Jefferson were given the task of creating a seal for the United States of America. It was finalized and approved six years later, on June 20, 1782. The Great Seal of the United States has the bald eagle in the center. A scroll car-ries the Latin words, E Pluribus Unum, meaning "out of many, one." This signifies one nation from thirteen colonies. In one claw, the eagle holds olive branches signifying the power of peace; in the other, a bundle of thirteen arrows signifying the power of war.

Above the eagle's head is a cloud surrounding a blue field containing thirteen stars, which forms a constellation. The constellation denotes a new state taking its place among other nations. Both sides of the Great Seal of the United States can be seen on the back of a one-dollar bill.

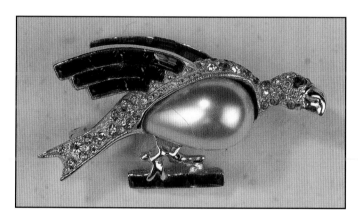

Fabulous eagle pin. Pearl body with red and blue baguette stones. Signed "Alvaire". 1940s.

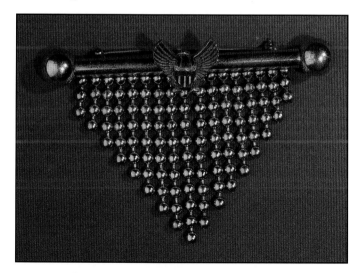

Gold pin with eagle and gold ball chain lengths. Eagle with enameled shield. Unsigned. 1940s.

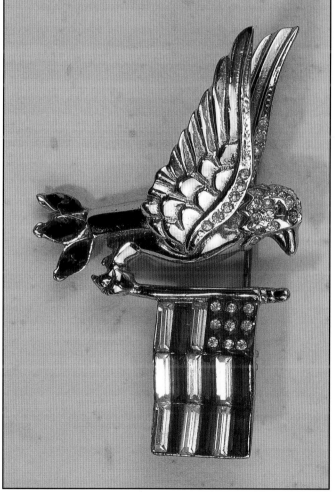

Pin of eagle carrying an American flag. Sterling, by Coro Craft. 1940.

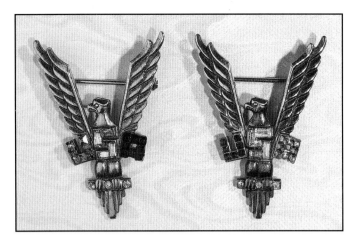

Two gold eagle pins with USA across the breast of the birds. Unsigned. 1940s.

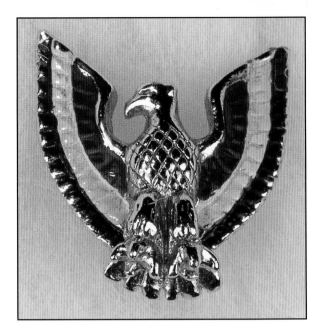

Very tiny eagle pin in red, white, and blue colors. Tie tack. 1-2" x 5-8". By Swank. 1960s.

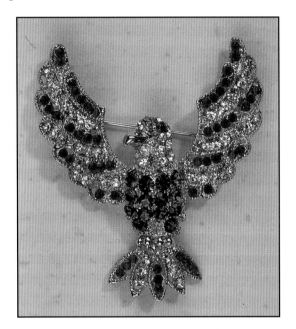

Eagle pin with red, clear, and blue rhinestones. Unsigned. Contemporary.

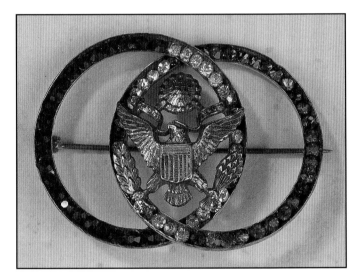

Pin with Great Seal eagle and two intertwined circles. WWII period.

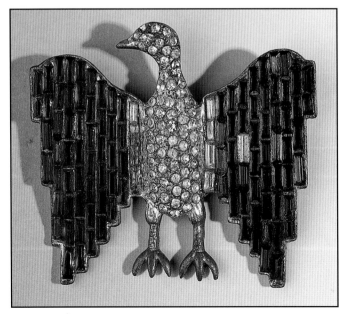

Eagle in red, clear, and blue rhinestones. Courtesy of Barbara Trujillo.

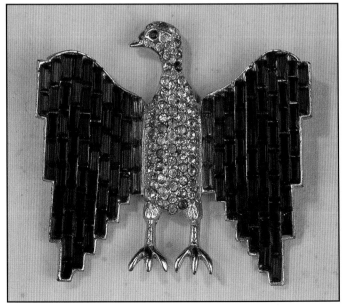

Pin of eagle in red baguette stones and clear rhinestones. Unsigned. WWII period.

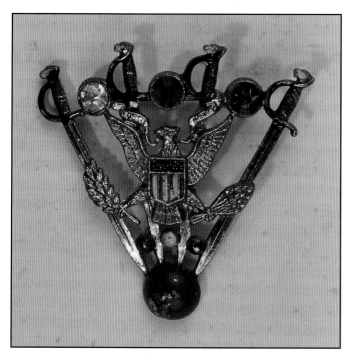

Pin with eagle and shield in the center and swords. Unsigned. WWII period.

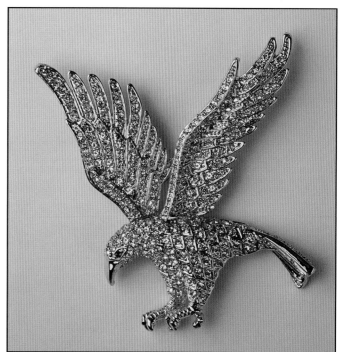

Large flying eagle pin of gold colored metal pave set with clear rhinestones and a green eye, 4-1-2" high. Unsigned. Contemporary.

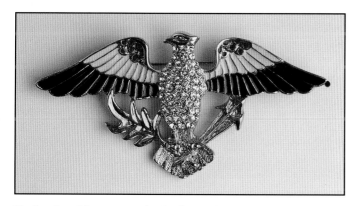

Eagle pin with outstretched wings of gold metal with red, white and blue enamel and pave rhinestone body, marked Eisenberg Ice ©.

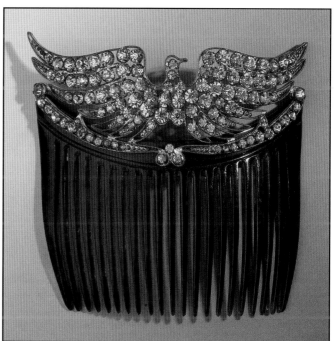

Eagle hair comb. 4 3-8" wing span. World War 1 period.

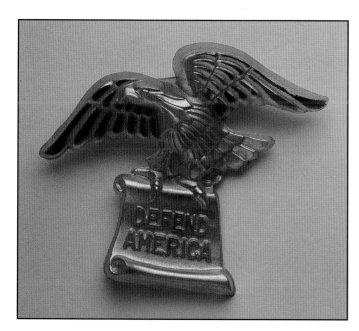

Cast pearlized white plastic pin of an eagle above a scroll lettered "DEFEND AMERICA". 1940s.

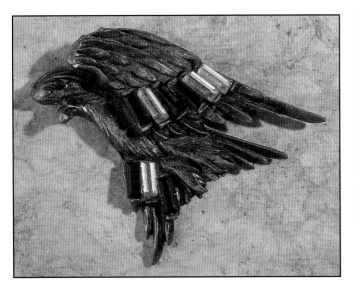

Eagle pin with red, white, and blue theme. Unsigned. 1940s.

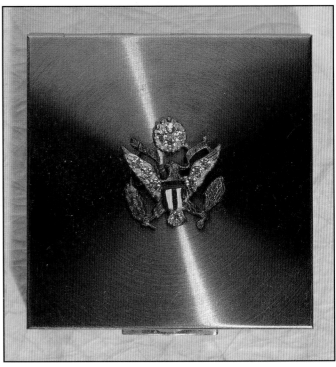

Compact with rhinestone pin on cover. World War II period.

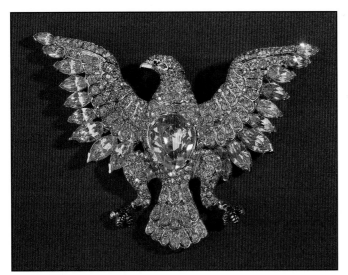

Silver eagle pin. Signed by Eisenberg. 4" wing span.

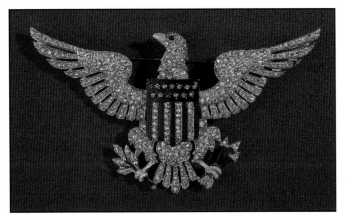

Eagle and American shield pin. Yellow feet. Signed Trifari.

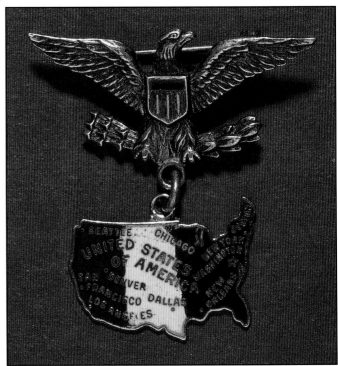

Cast eagle pin with American shield and a pendant map of the United States in red, white, and blue enamel and lettering "United States of America" and the names and locations of 10 major cities. Back marked "God Bless America, Wells Ster." 1970s.

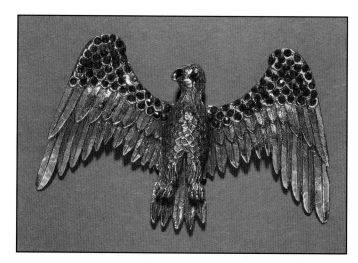

Gold metal eagle pendant-pin with red rhinestones. Unmarked. 1970s.

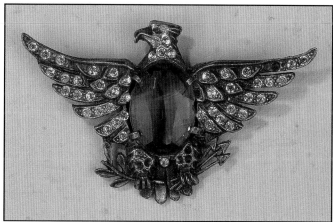

Gold metal eagle pin with red, white, and blue rhinestones in the letters USA. Unmarked. 1960s.

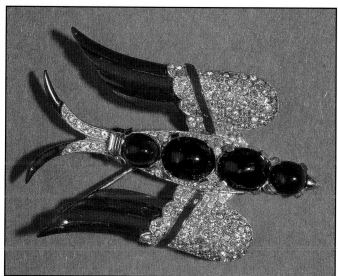

Eagle pin of red and blue oval cabochons, clear rhinestones, and red and blue enamel on cast pot metal. Unsigned. 1960s.

Majestic eagle pin with large blue rhinestone in the center. In his right talon, he grasps an olive branch, in his left talon, he grasps arrows, 1930s.

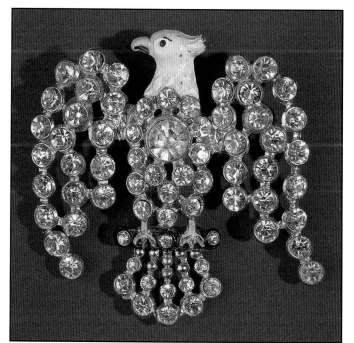

Eagle pin with clear round rhinestones. Courtesy of Barbara Trujillo.

Gold star pin with a two-headed eagle in the center. The two-headed eagle has been a patriotic symbol in Eastern Europe since the 15th century; the origin of this pin is unknown.

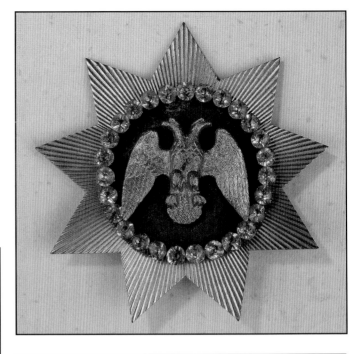

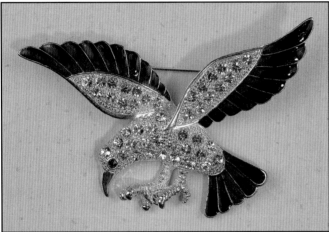

Large eagle pin with red and blue on the tips of wings and tail feathers. 4 5-8" wing to wing. Unsigned. Contemporary.

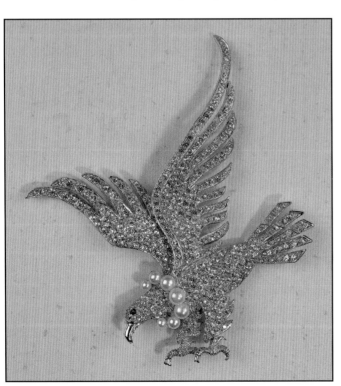

Dress clip of a copper, 5-pointed star curved around a gold metal disc with eagle and inscription "Friends Of New York State Soldiers, Sailors." The disc is mounted on a tapering metal band that is enameled as an American flag in red and white stripes and a blue field with 13 white stars. Marked "Cartier, U S Pat. 2-220-442." 1940s.

Large silver eagle pin with clear rhinestones and a pearl "necklace". 4" x 4 3-4". Unsigned. 1950s.

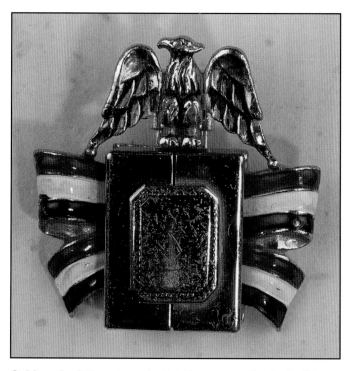

Gold eagle sitting atop a locket that opens. Patriotic ribbons on each side. Dress clip. WWII period.

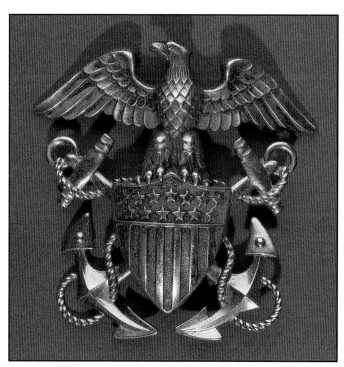

Eagle and shield pin. 2 1-2" square. 1940s.

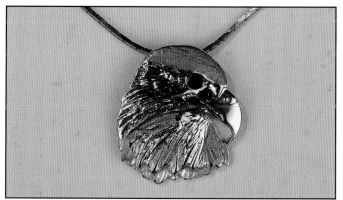

Gold necklace with eagle charm and red rhinestone eye. 1960s.

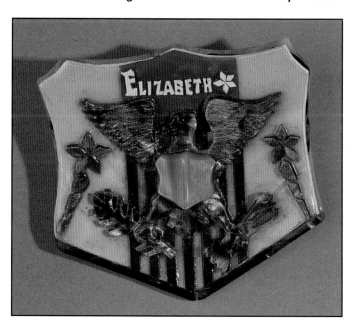

Eagle's head pin with red rhinestone for the eye and blue and clear rhinestones in feathers. Signed Trifari. Contemporary.

Layered plastic eagle on top of red and white stripes of flag with "Elizabeth" in blue part of flag. 1940s.

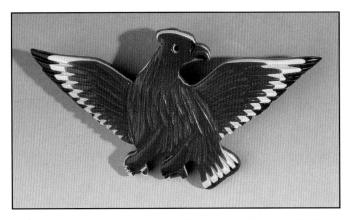

Red, white, and blue eagle pin. Courtesy of Barbara Trujillo.

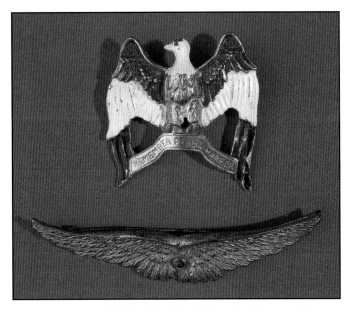

"Remember Pearl Harbor" eagle pin in red, white, and blue colors. Gold spread eagle's wings. Courtesy of Barbara Trujillo.

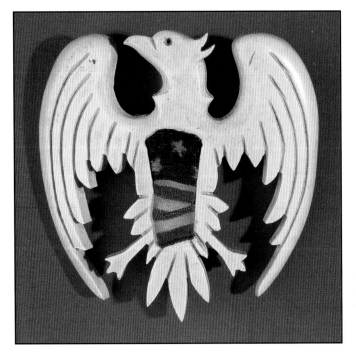

Early Bakelite eagle pin with lion, other animals on spread wings. 3 1-2" h x 2". 1940s.

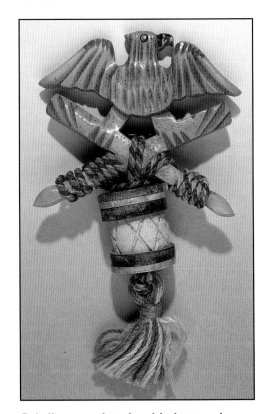

Bakelite carved eagle with drum and woven cord. 1940s.

White Bakelite eagle pin with partial fabric American flag in the center. 2 1-2" square. 1940s.

Gold eagle pin with black breast. Courtesy of Barbara Trujillo.

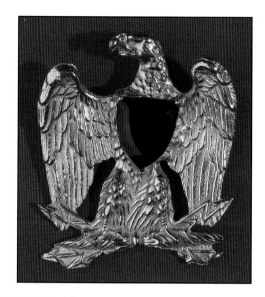

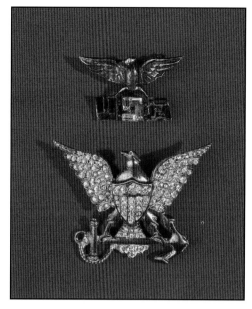

Eagle sitting atop the letters "USA". Eagle pin in gold and clear rhinestones holding an anchor in its claws. Courtesy of Barbara Trujillo.

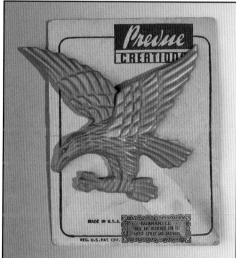

Green eagle pin. Courtesy of Barbara Trujillo.

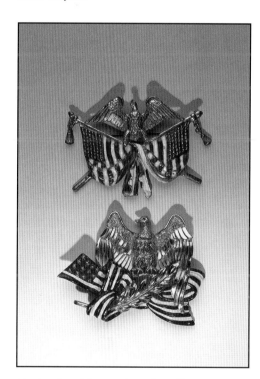

Eagle pin with two American flags crossed at the poles. Eagle pin with American flag tied up like a bow. Courtesy of Barbara Trujillo.

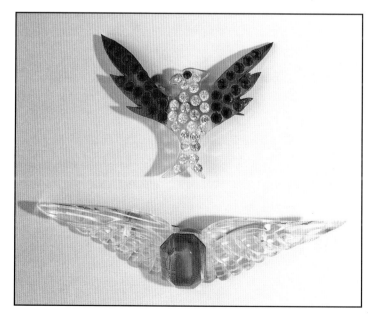

Eagle pin in red, white, and blue rhinestones. Spread eagle wings pin with blue stone center. Courtesy of Barbara Trujillo.

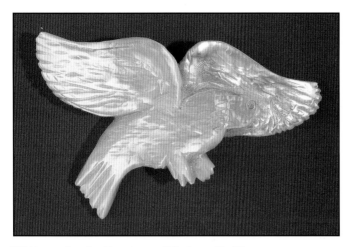

White eagle pin. Courtesy of Barbara Trujillo.

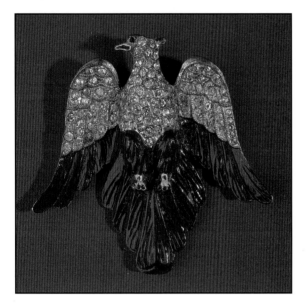

Eagle pin in black and clear rhinestones. Courtesy of Barbara Trujillo.

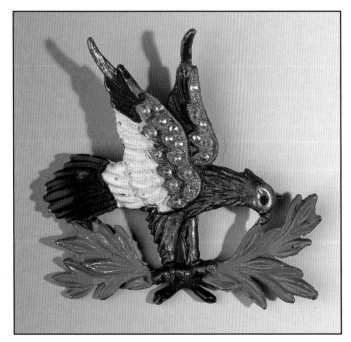

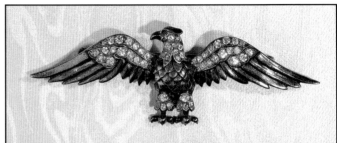

Eagle pin in red, white, and blue. Signed Trifari.

Small gold eagle pin with clear rhinestones. Signed Trifari.

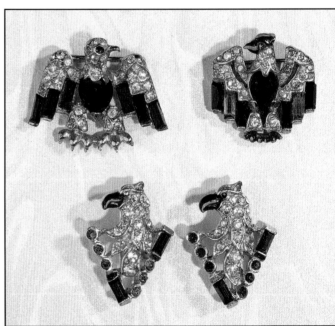

Four small pins, pair of eagles and pair of eagles in the center of V. All signed Trifari.

Silver, red, white, and blue eagle pin. Courtesy of Barbara Trujillo.

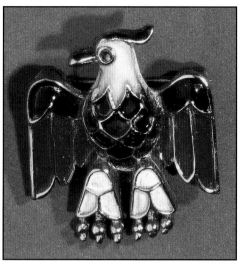

Small red, white, and blue eagle pin.
Signed Trifari. Contemporary.

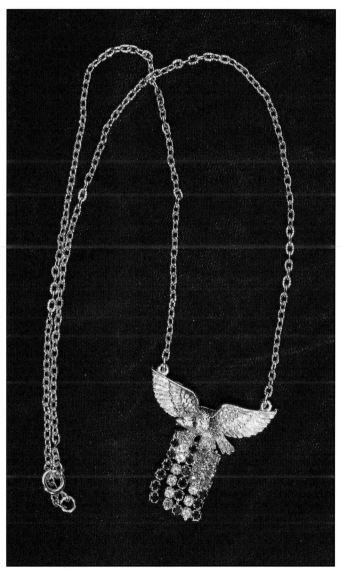

Soaring gold eagle pin with red, clear, and blue rhinestones
by Napier. Contemporary.

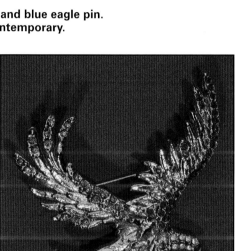

Gold eagle
pin with
rhinestones.
Unsigned.
Contemporary.

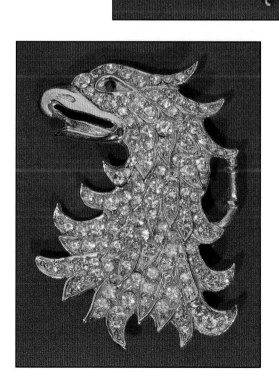

Gold chain necklace with eagle and patriotic rhinestones
pendant. Unmarked. 1960s.

Gold eagle head with clear rhinestones
belt buckle. Contemporary.

Gold eagle pin with red rhinestones. Signed Kramer of New York.

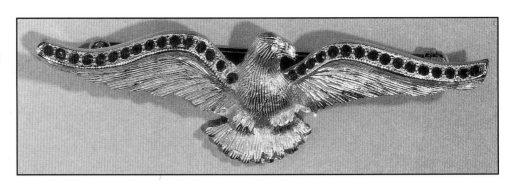

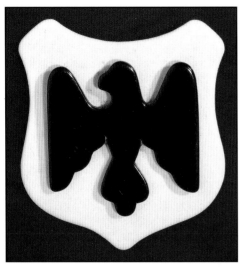

Shield pin with black plastic eagle on white plastic background. 1960s.

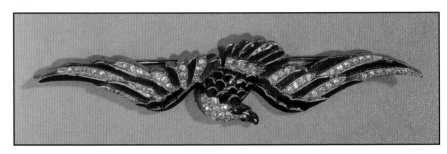

Soaring eagle pin in patriotic colors. Signed by Trifari.

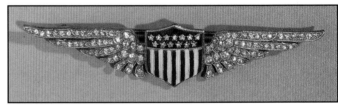

Wings of the eagle and American flag shield in enamel and rhinestones. Trifari.

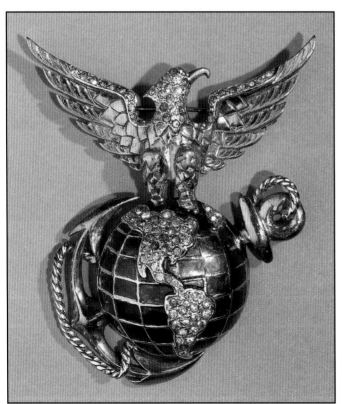

Pin with eagle sitting atop the earth with an anchor.

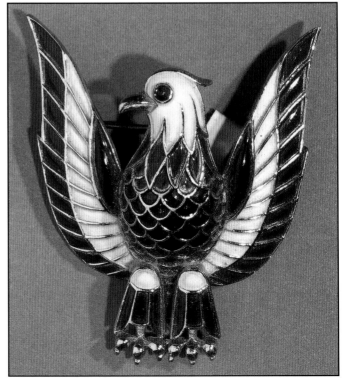

Eagle pin in red, white, and blue enamel. By Trifari. Contemporary.

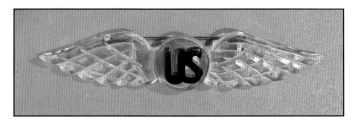

Lucite pin with black US letters in the center of spread eagle's wings. 1940s.

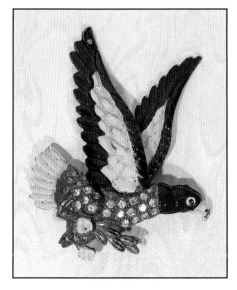

Eagle pin in red, white, and blue enamels and rhinestones. Unsigned. 1940s.

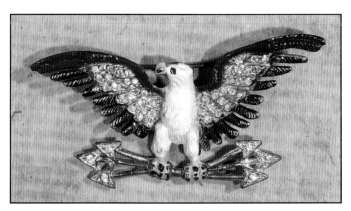

Eagle pin in red, white, and blue enamel and clear rhinestones, carrying arrows in yellow feet. Unsigned. 1940s.

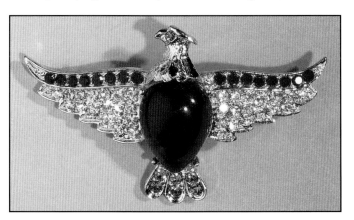

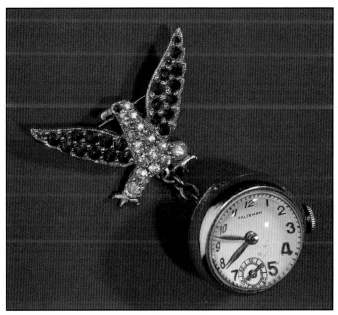

Silver and rhinestone eagle pin with shield. Ribbon marked "E Pluribus Unum" Unsigned. 1940.

Silver eagle watch pin. marked "Talisman." 1940s.

Silver eagle pin with large red cabochon rhinestone in center. Unsigned. 1940s.

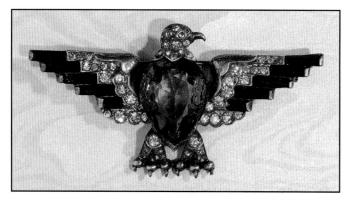

Silver eagle pin with large blue faceted rhinestone in center. Marked sterling. 1940s.

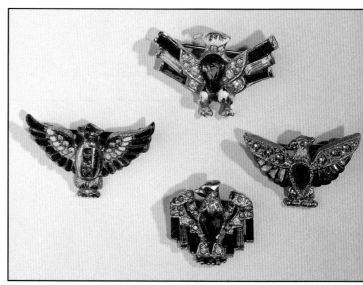

4 assorted eagle pins with patriotic colors. Left, sterling by Coro. Bottom with indistinct letters #220, others unmarked.

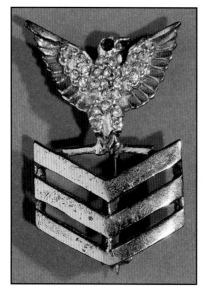

Gold eagle pin with red eye and emblem with 3 bars. Marked sterling.

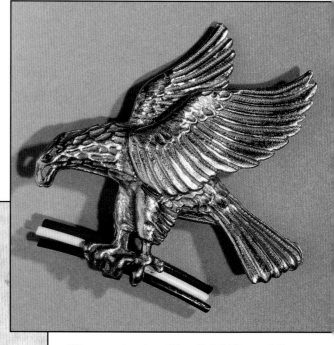

Silver eagle pin with celluloid lines at the bottom. Unsigned. 1940s.

3 assorted eagle pins with patriotic enameled colors. Marked Coro. 1940s.

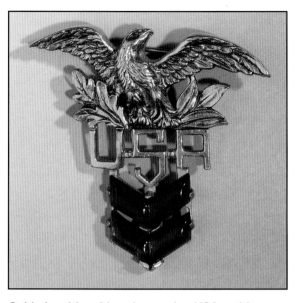

Gold pin with gold eagle carrying USA emblem.

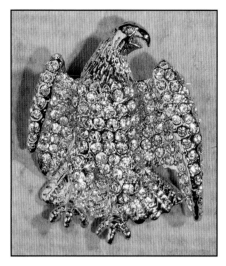

Gold eagle pin with clear rhinestones. Unsigned. 1950s.

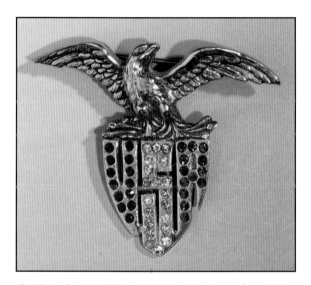

Gold eagle and USA shield pin. Unsigned. c. 1950s.

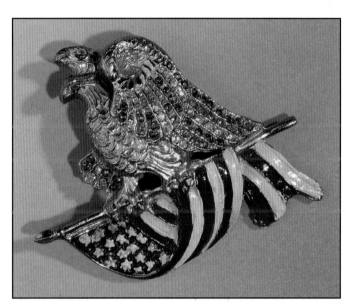

Gold eagle with red, clear, and blue rhinestones carrying an American flag. Unsigned. 1940s.

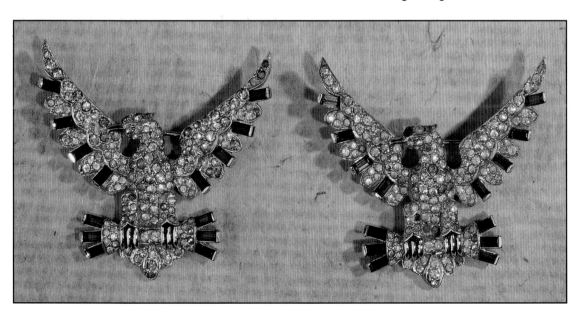

Two silver eagle pins with varied colored rhinestones by Mazer, 1940s.

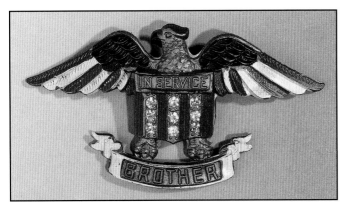

Gold plastic eagle in patriotic enameled colors carrying a banner that reads "In Service" "Brother".

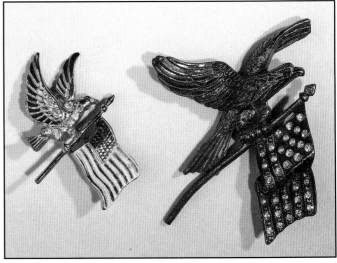

Two gold flying eagle pins, both carrying the American flag. Unsigned. 1940s.

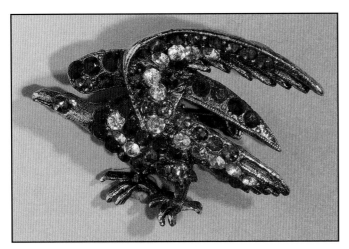

Eagle pin with red, clear, and blue rhinestones. Unsigned. 1940s.

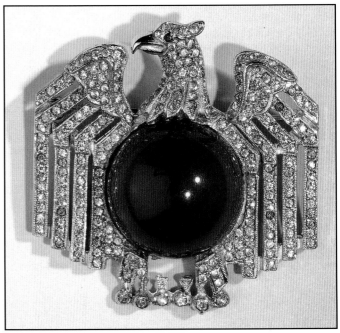

Silver eagle pin with red eye and red cabochon center stone. Unsigned. 1940s.

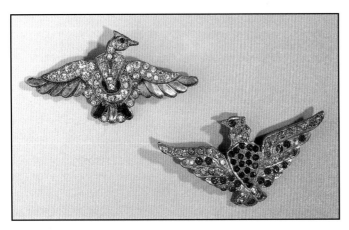

Two eagle pins, one in gold, the other in silver with patriotic colored rhinestones. Unsigned. 1940s.

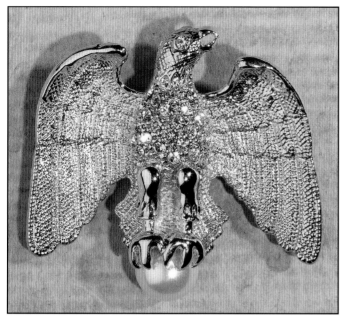

Silver and gold eagle pin with pearl. Gold stripe. Unsigned. 1960s.

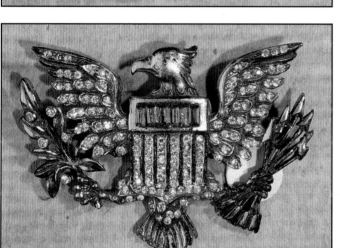

Eagle pin with red, white, and blue stripes, arrows, and olive branch. Unsigned. 1940s.

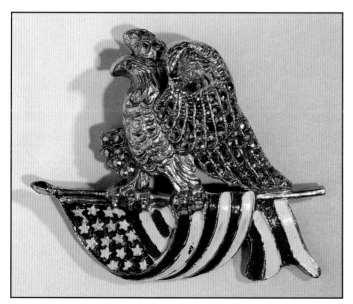

Gold plastic eagle pin with red eye carrying arrows and olive branch. Unsigned. 1940s.

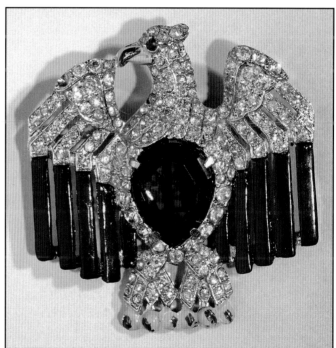

Eagle pin in patriotic theme. Blue faceted belly, enameled wing tips, yellow feet and beak. Unsigned. 1940s.

Silver marcasite eagle carrying enameled American Flag pin. Unsigned. 1940s.

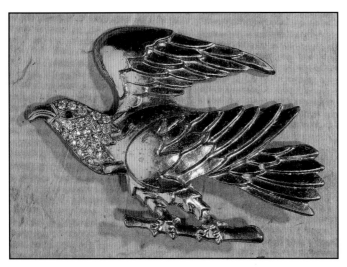

Gold flying eagle pin with red eye. Unsigned. 1940s.

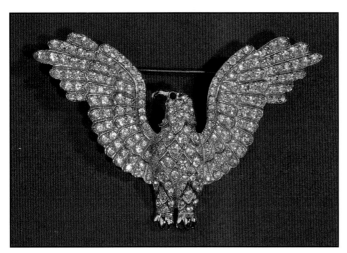

Silver eagle pin. All clear stones. By Coro. 1950s.

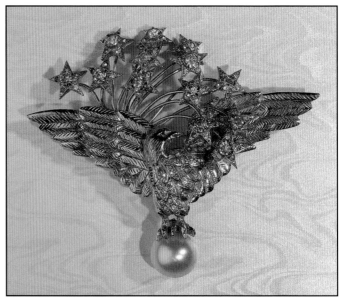

Spectacular gold pin with an eagle, stars, and a pearl drop. 4" wingspan. Signed Eisenberg.

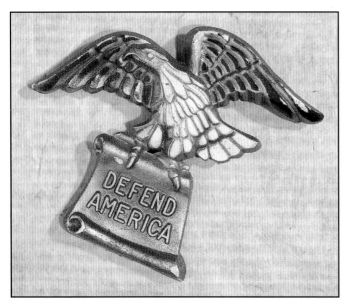

Plastic pin with red, white, and blue eagle carrying a scroll that reads "Defend America". 1940s.

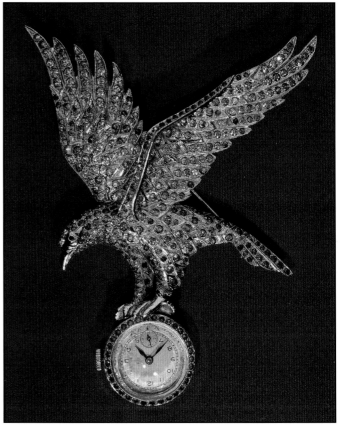

Silver eagle pin with marcasite carrying a watch face. 3 1-2" tall. c. 1940s,

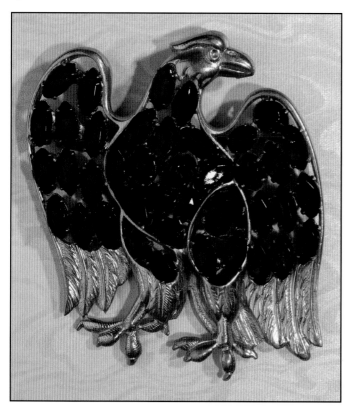

Gold and red eagle pin, signed Hattie Carnegie. Sterling. 3" x 2 1-2". c. 1940s.

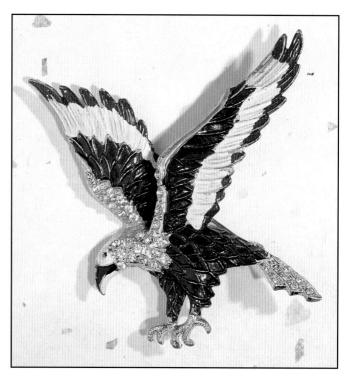

Eagle pin painted in patriotic colors. Dated 1930.

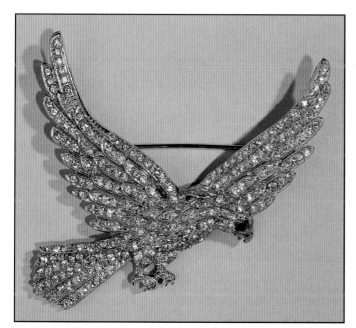

Pin of silver eagle with red eye. Unsigned. 1940s.

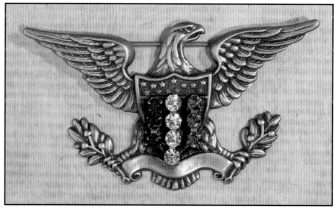

Gold eagle pin with red, white, and blue striped crest. Signed Joseff of Hollywood.

Silver eagle with red, white, and blue colors grasping an olive branch and arrows. Unsigned. c. 1940s.

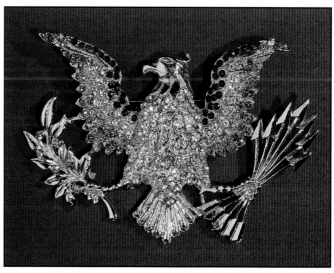

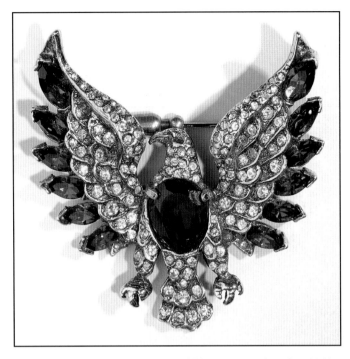

Eagle pin, faceted red stone and blue stone wing tips 1940s.

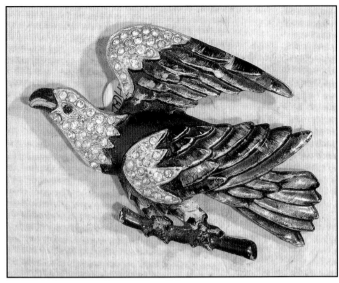

Eagle pin in red and clear stones and blue enamel. Unsigned. c. 1940s.

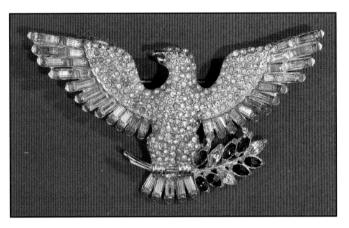

Silver and rhinestone pin of an eagle holding an olive branch with blue, red, and clear stones. Unsigned. c. 1940s.

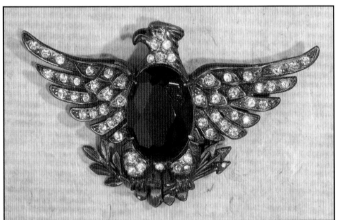

Eagle pin, with red faceted stone, grasping in it's claws an olive branch and arrows . 1930s.

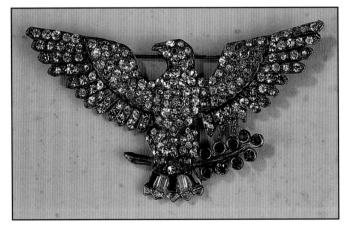

Another variation of a rhinestone eagle pin with colored stones in the olive branch and tail. Unsigned. 1940s.

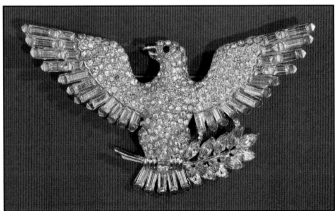

Silver and rhinestone pin of an eagle with a red eye holding an olive branch. Unsigned. 1940s.

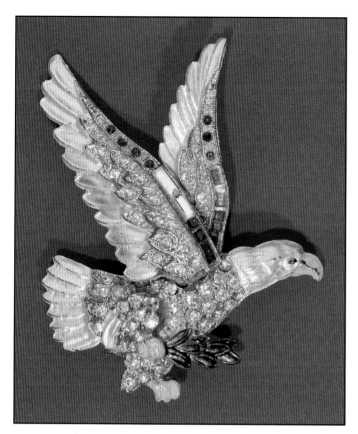

Eagle pin with red, white, and blue rhinestones holding an olive branch. Yellow enamel beak and feet and white wing tips. Unsigned. c. 1940s.

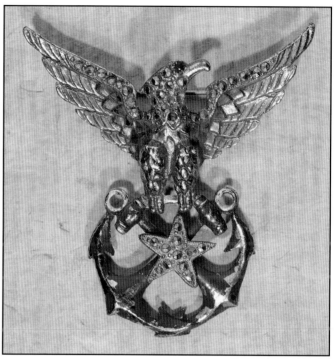

Silver eagle pin with a red eye grasping two red enameled anchors in it's claws. Unsigned. 1940s.,

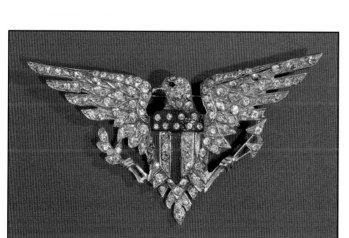

Silver eagle pin with American shield holding arrows and olive branch. Unsigned. 1940s.

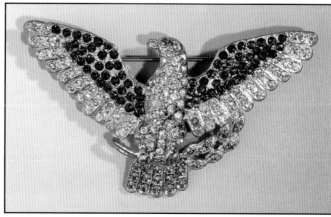

Eagle pin with red, white, and blue stones. Unsigned. 1940s.

Wildlife

Many Americans especially love animals, so it is that animals and patriotism are often combined. Many different animals have been included in red, white and blue jewelry, from cats and bears to turtles and butterflies. Of course, American artist Walt Disney's beloved Mickey Mouse is among the menagerie!

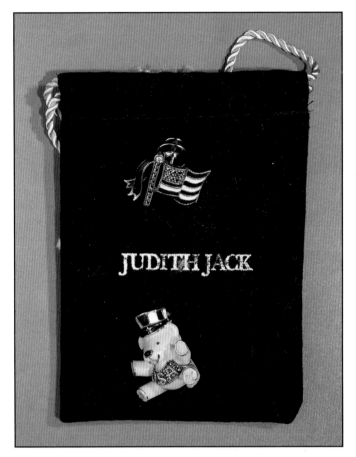

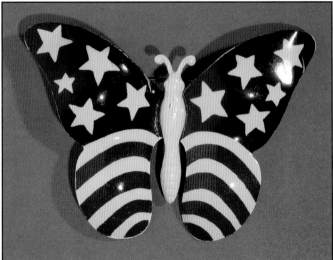

Butterfly pin with wings that represent the American flag. Celluloid. 1960s.

2 pins by Judith Jack enameled with marcasite. Contemporary.

Gold choker necklace with butterfly in center in patriotic colors. 1960s.

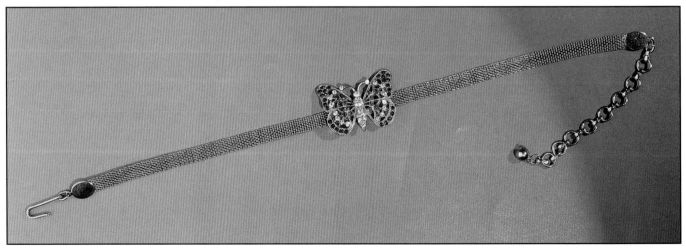

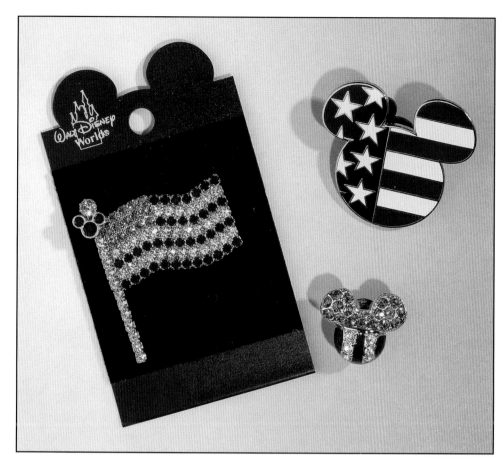

Walt Disney World American flag pin, Mickey Mouse head pin representing American flag, and another smaller Mickey Mouse pin in red, clear, and blue rhinestones. Contemporary.

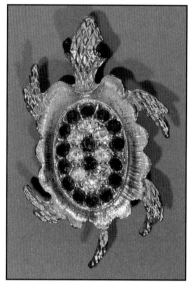

Gold turtle pin with red, clear, and blue rhinestones. Contemporary.

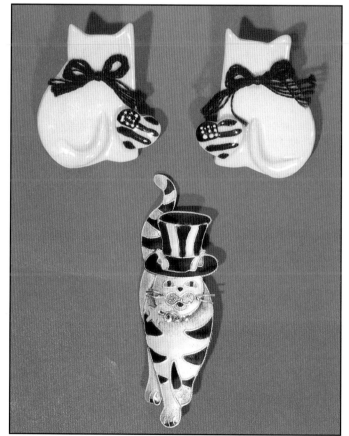

Three cats in American flag theme; a pair of earrings and a pin. Unsigned. Contemporary.

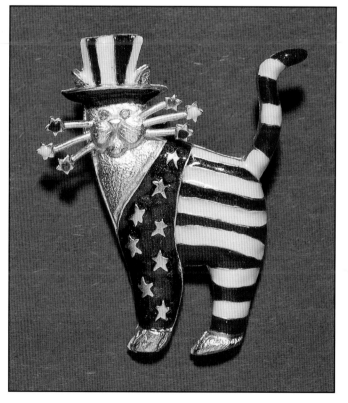

Cast white metal cat pin dressed in red, white and blue enamel flag-design clothing, and stars on his whiskers. Unmarked. Contemporary.

Dated Events

Many significant events in American history have been immortalized in patriotic jewelry.

The Liberty Bell is a symbol of freedom in the United States. It rang out when the Continental Congress signed the Declaration of Independence in 1776. The Bicentennial of 1976 remembered this.

The Liberty Bell was cast in London, England, in 1752. The bell cracked when it was tolled during the funeral procession of the United States' first Supreme Court chief justice, John Marshall. A new bell was made from the metal in the old one. This one also cracked, and a third bell was built from the same metal. It was first called The Liberty Bell by abolitionist publications in the 1830s. The bell thereafter was adopted as a symbol of liberty to promote a wide variety of causes, from women's rights to civil rights to protests against political oppression.

Japan's military air attack on Pearl Harbor in Honolulu, Hawaii, on December 7, 1941, fueled a determination for America to join in the military action of World War Two. The popular quote, "Remember Pearl Harbor" reflects this sentiment and was the slogan that rallied the nation and inspired jewelry of this period.

The United States' astronauts successfully landed on the moon in 1969. Americans were proud of the achievement.

Even moments of horrific tragedy for our nation, such as the terrorist attacks on the World Trade Center in New York, on the Pentagon in Virginia, and the crash of a hijacked plane in Pennsylvania, on September 11, 2001, are commemorated with especially designed items.

Patriotic jewelry reflects deep personal feelings that "We Will Not Forget!"

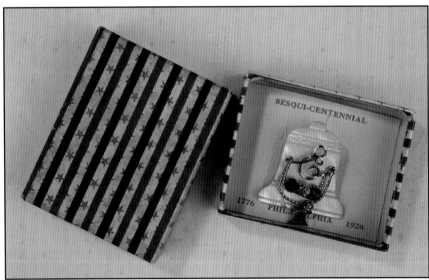

The sesqui-centennial celebrations in Philadelphia in 1926 inspired this Liberty Bell pin with its original box.

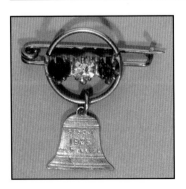

Tiny gold Liberty bell pin with red, clear, and blue rhinestone. Unsigned. 1940s.

Liberty Bell pin. Unsigned. 1940s.

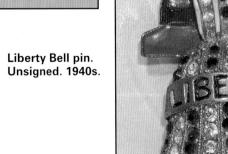

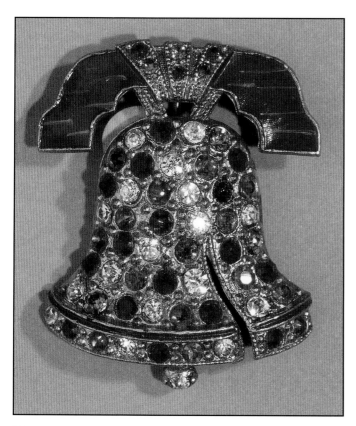

Liberty Bell pin in gold metal and rhinestones. Unsigned. 1940s.

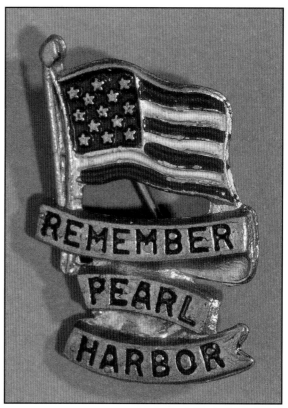

"Remember Pearl Harbor" pin with American flag. 1940s.

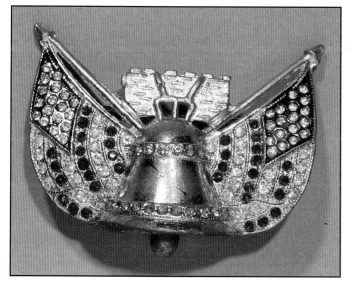

Liberty bell and two American flags on either side with red, clear, and blue rhinestones. 1940s.

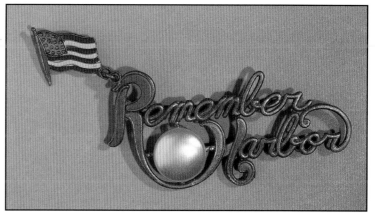

"Remember Pearl Harbor" pin with American flag. 1940s.

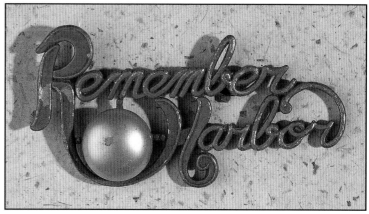

Remember Pearl Harbor pin. 1940s.

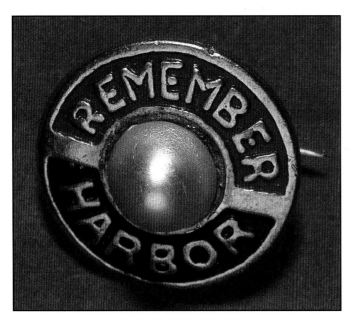

Lapel pin of stamped metal with enamel and central pearl. The frame reads "Remember   Harbor." Unmarked. 1940s.

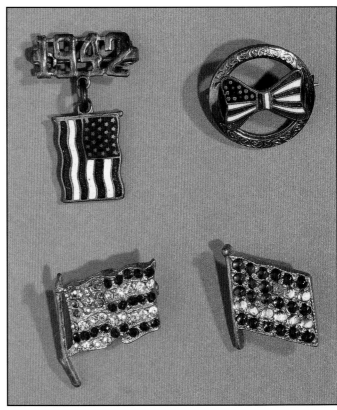

"1942" pin with American flag dangling. Enameled metal pin with bow in red, white, and blue. Two American flag pins with red, clear, and blue rhinestones. The bottom right pin is marked Enco.

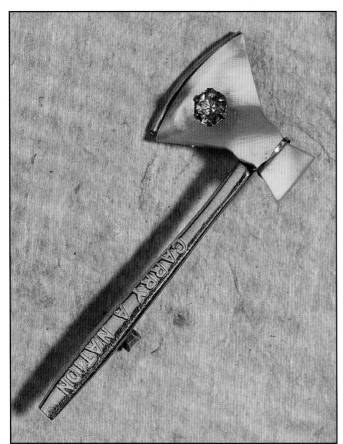

Gold metal and mother-of-pearl HOME DEFENDER hatchet pin with a faceted rhinestone and white enamel reading "CARRY A. NATION." 1940s.

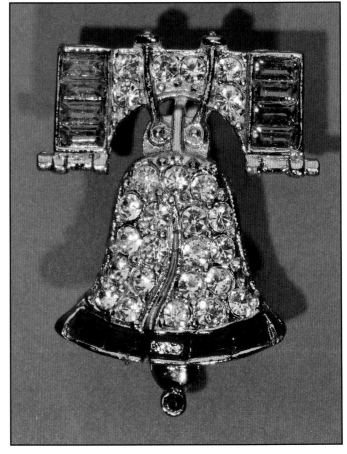

Liberty Bell pin. 1960s.

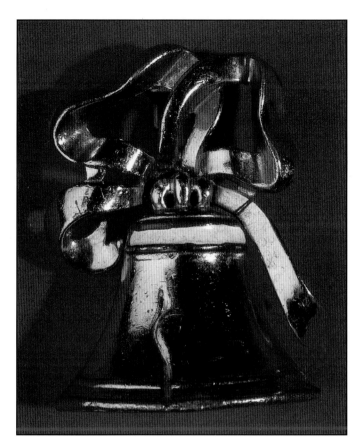

Gold Liberty Bell with ribbon on top. Courtesy of Barbara Trujillo.

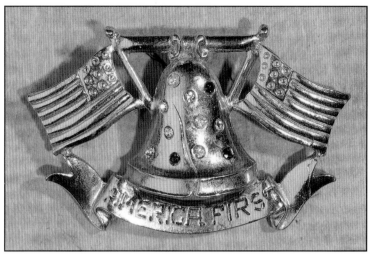

Gold "America First" pin has flags on either side of bell. Unsigned. 1960s.

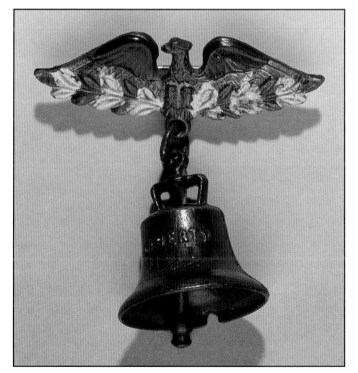

Eagle grasping the Liberty Bell. Courtesy of Barbara Trujillo.

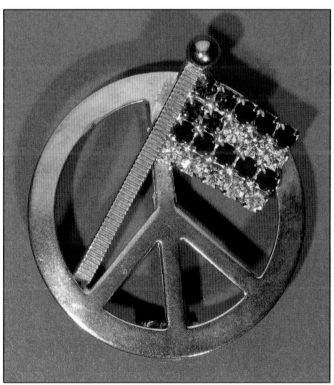

Silver pin with American flag and peace symbol in the center. 1960s.

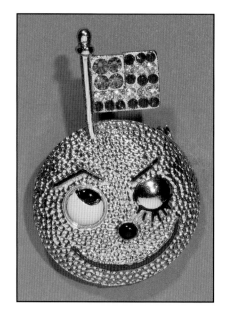

American flag commemorating man landing on the moon. July 20, 1969. Unsigned.

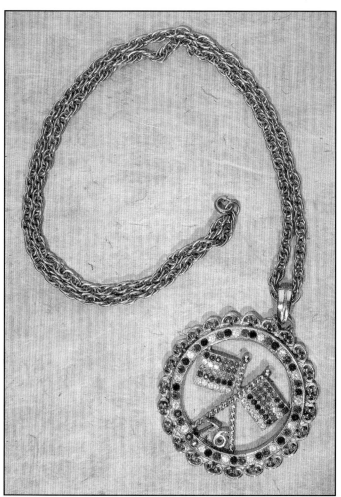

Gold necklace has emblem of two American flags and "76". 1976.

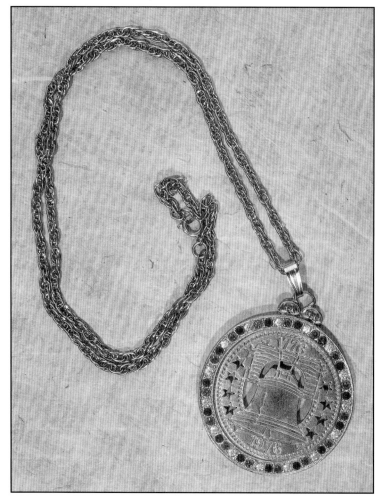

Bicentennial necklace with Liberty Bell disc and red, clear, and blue rhinestones surrounding it. 1976.

Two necklaces with "76" in a circle emblem. 1976.

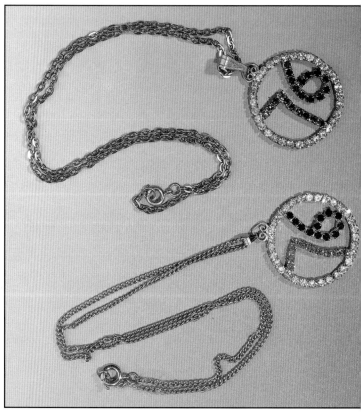

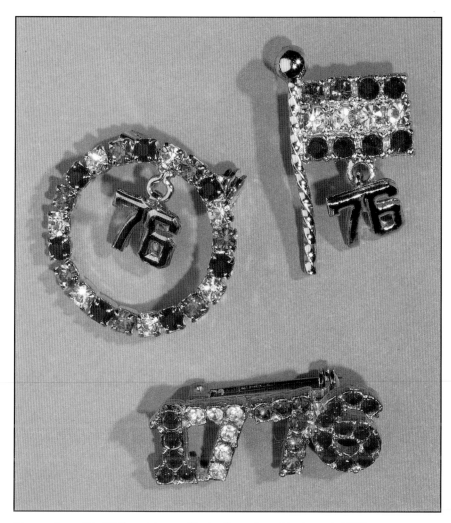

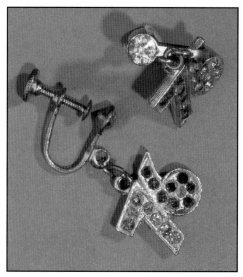

Bicentennial dangling earrings with "76" emblems.

Three pins with "76" emblems. Circle, flag, date. Unsigned. 1976.

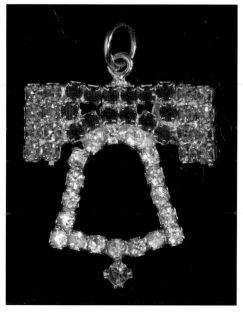

Rhinestone charm in the form of a bell. 1976.

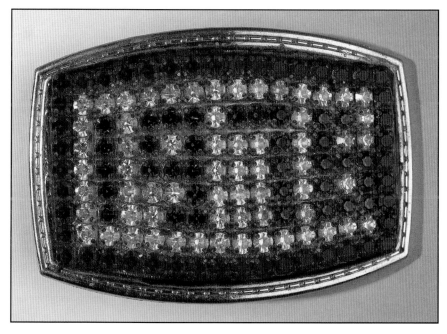

Bicentennial belt buckle with red, clear, and blue rhinestones. 1976.

Liberty bell pin in red and white rhinestones. 1940s.

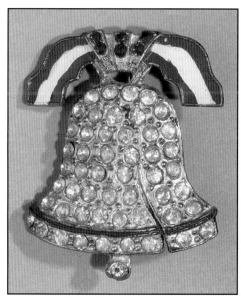

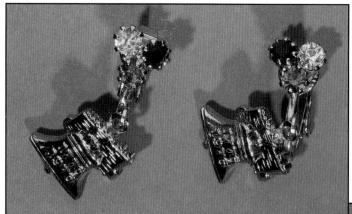

Bicentennial Liberty
bell dangling earrings.
1976.

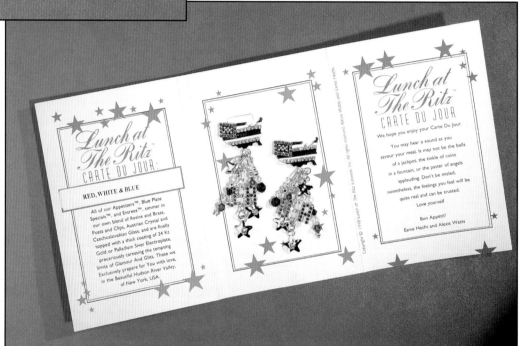

Lunch at the Ritz Carte
Du Jour flyer with a pair
of flags and star pen-
dent earrings. Contem-
porary.

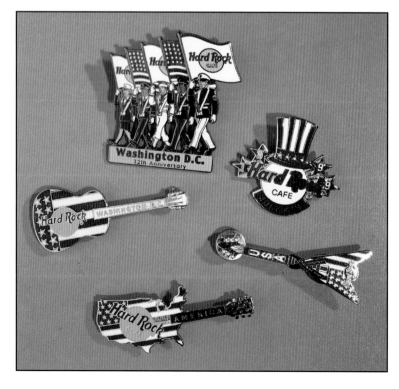

Assorted Hard Rock Cafe
pins. 1980s-'90s.

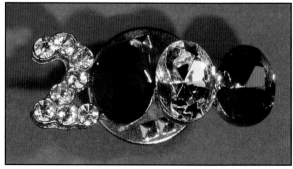

Gold pin with red, clear, and blue rhinestones. 2000.

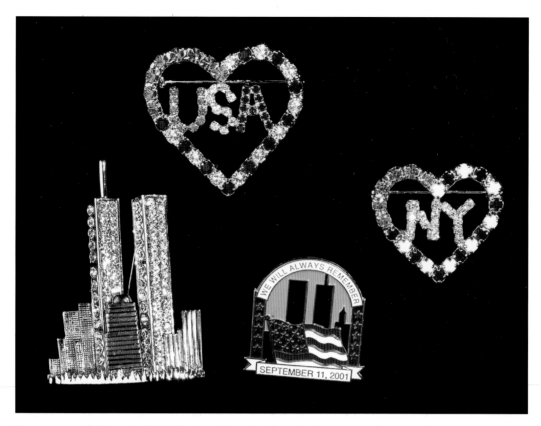

Four assorted pins, the Twin Towers, New York, and USA representing the tragedy of September 11, 2001. The NY and USA hearts are signed Bauer.

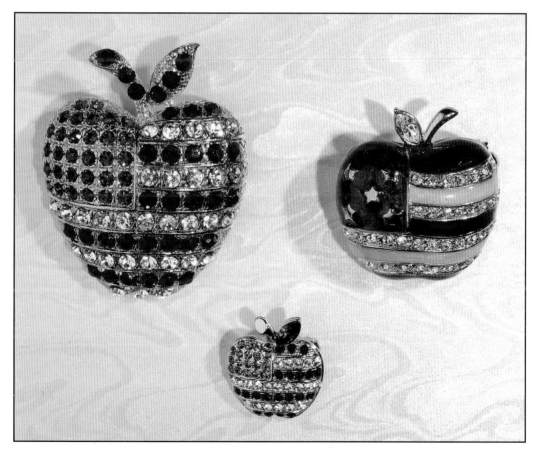

Three pins in apple shapes with American flag colored rhinestones, all contemporary. Marked "9-11-2001." Unsigned.

Christmas

Much of the patriotic Christmas jewelry that can be found today is of recent date. Some fabulous designer jewelry has been created for patriotic Christmas elves!

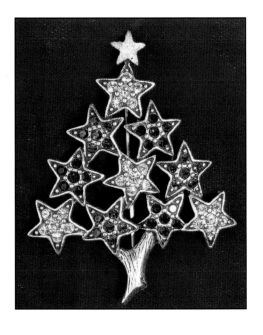

Stars forming the shape of a Christmas tree with red, clear, and blue rhinestones. Unsigned. Contemporary.

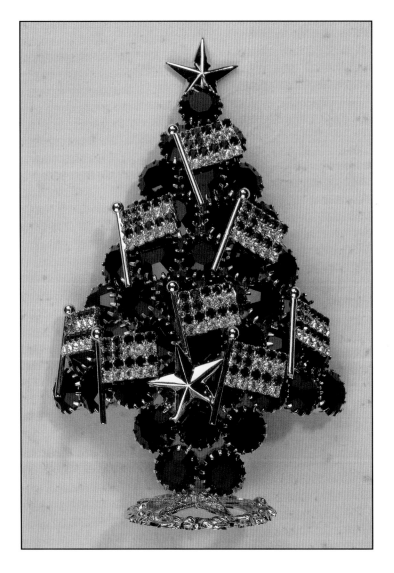

Black Christmas tree pin with American flags and stars. Made by Anthony Attruia to commemorate 9-11-2001. 4 3/4" tall.

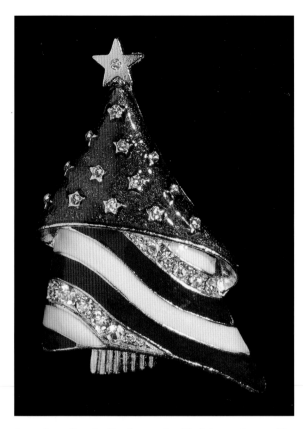

American flag in the form of a Christmas tree with gold star. "Remember 9-11-2001" Linea M USA.

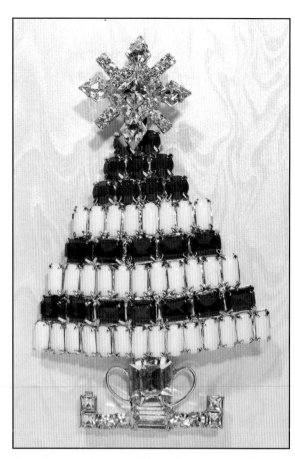

Pin with red, clear, and blue rhinestones and white opaque stones. Star on top, signed Lawrence Vrba, 4 1/4" tall.

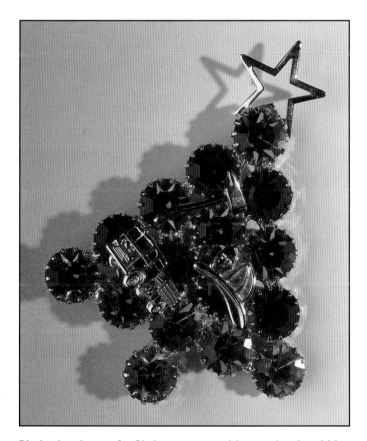

Pin in the shape of a Christmas tree with round red and blue rhinestones with a star sitting atop. 3" tall by Anthony Attruia. As a tribute to the firemen of 9-11-01.

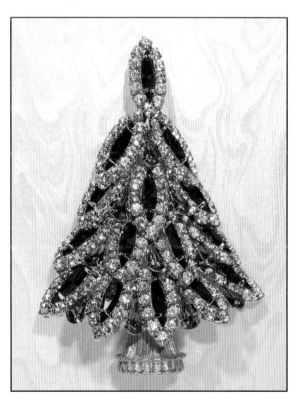

Limited edition Christmas tree pin with red, clear, and blue rhinestones, numbers on back "12/120, 12-1-2001", 3 1/2"h.

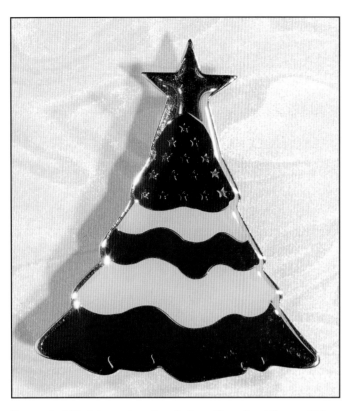

Enameled Christmas tree lapel pin with red, white, and blue colors and gold star on top. Unsigned. Contemporary.

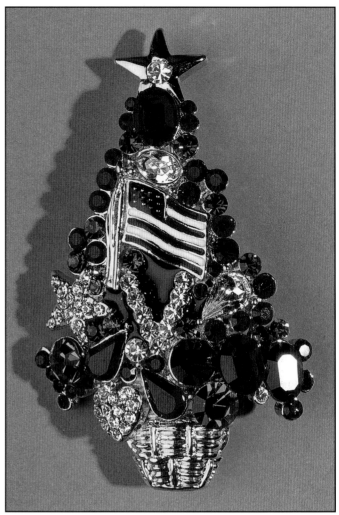

Christmas tree pin with American flag decoration. Marked OTC.

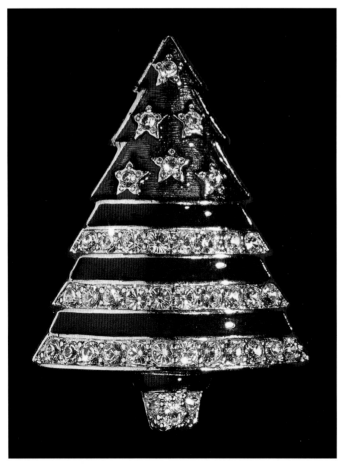

Christmas tree pin in red and blue enamel and clear rhinestones. By contemporary designer Christopher Radko.

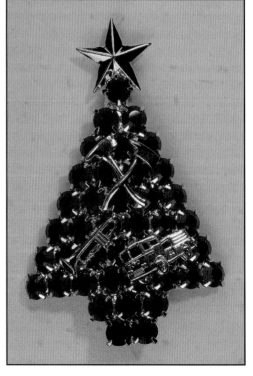

Christmas tree pin with red rhinestones and gold star atop, decorated with a fire engine, bugle, and axes. This was made by Anthony Attruia as a tribute to the firefighters of 9-11-2001.

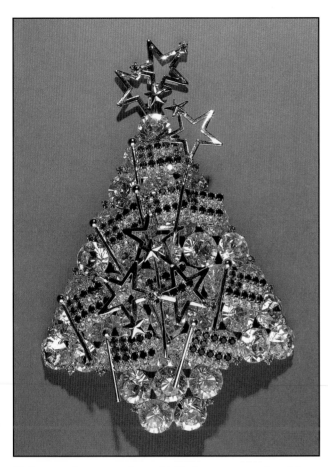

Unique and spectacular gold Christmas tree pin with stars and flags for decoration. Swarovski crystals and 14k gold wash on the stars. Made by Anthony Attruia especially for Richard Silverman. 5" tall.

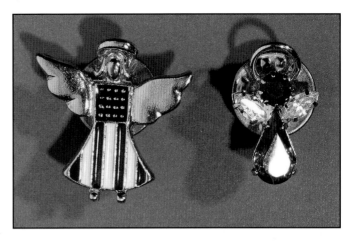

Enameled pin with angel. Another angel pin with red, clear, and blue rhinestones. Marked USA. Contemporary.

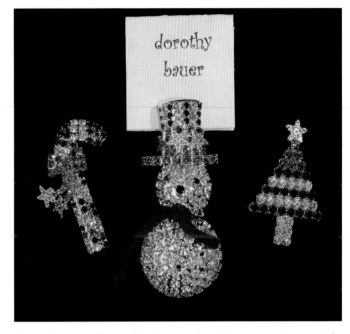
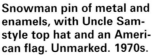

Three Dorothy Bauer Christmas pins in contemporary candy cane, snowman, and Christmas tree shapes.

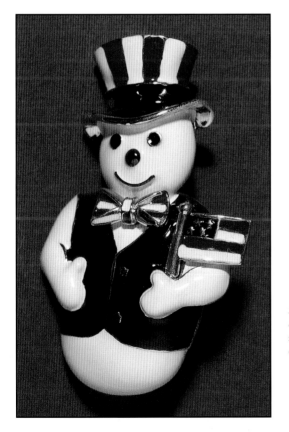

Enameled composition snowman wearing patriotic hat from Enesco, designed by Linda Lindquist Baldwin. "From a nickel to a snow snickel".

Snowman pin of metal and enamels, with Uncle Sam-style top hat and an American flag. Unmarked. 1970s.

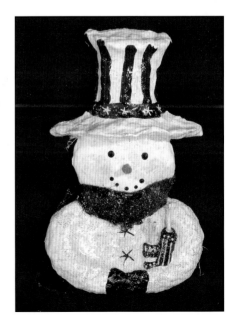

Say It In Words

Words are powerful; they create as well as reflect our thoughts. Names in red, white, and blue can show patriotism.

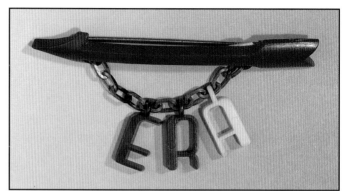

Plastic pin with ERA initials. 1940s.

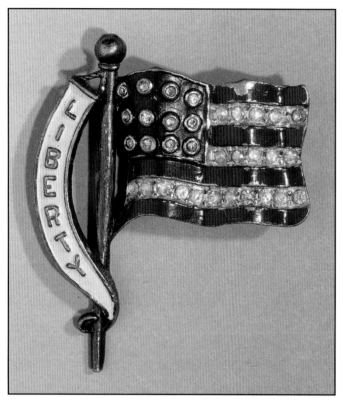

Waving American flag pin with a banner reading "Liberty". 1930s

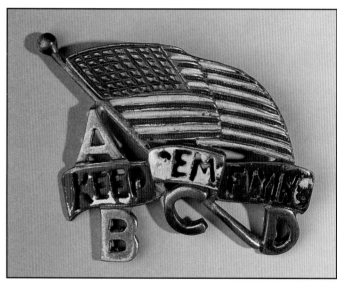

"Keep 'Em Flying" banner on American flag. Courtesy of Barbara Trujillo.

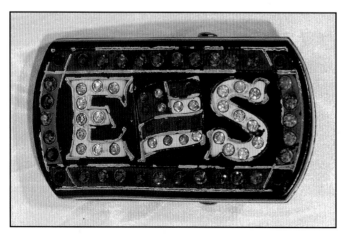

Pin with blue, green, red, and clear rhinestones with "ES" and American flag in the center. Layered belt buckle. This has my late sister's initials.

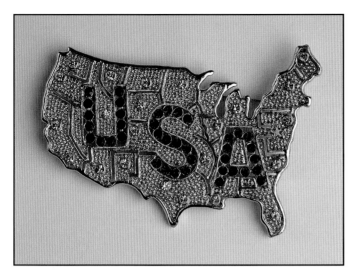

Silver metal map of the United States with red, blue and puple rhinestones spelling USA, and the boundaries of the states cut out, with a pierced star at the Washington, DC. location. 3 1/8" wide.

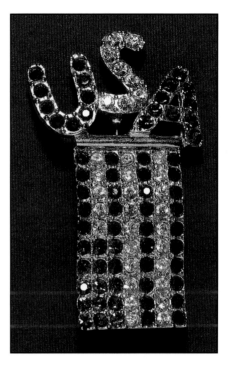

Pin of rhinestones and gold washed metal with letters USA and American flag. 1970s.

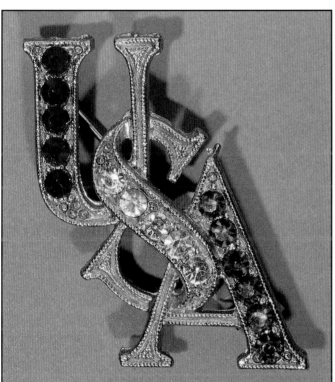

Gold USA pin with red, clear, and blue rhinestones. Unsigned. Contemporary.

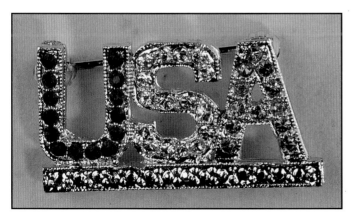

Pin with "USA" in red, clear, and blue rhinestones. Unsigned. Contemporary.

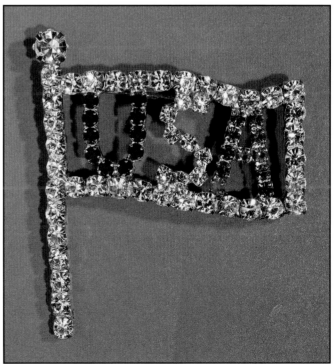

Flag pin with USA rhinestone letters inside. Contemporary.

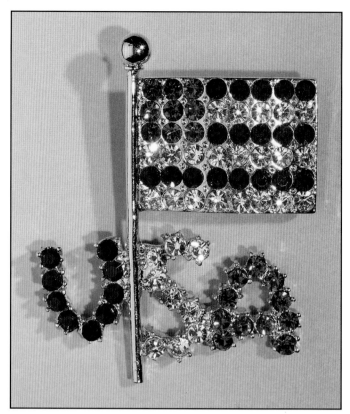

American flag and USA pin in gold and red, clear, and blue rhinestones. Unmarked. Contemporary.

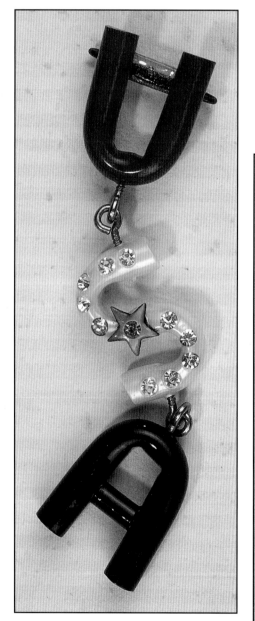

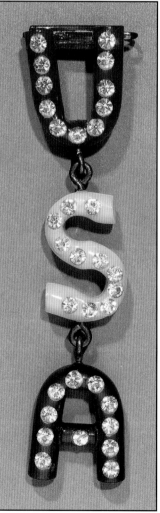

Dangling USA Bakelite pin in red, white, and blue colors with clear rhinestones. 1940s.

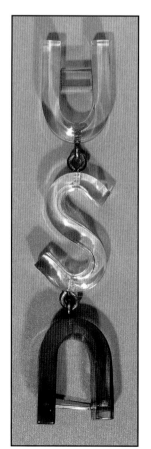

Dangling USA Lucite pin.

Pin with dangling USA letters. Bakelite. A bit different with the star and rhinestones on the "S". WWII period.

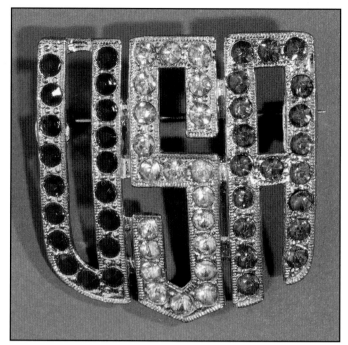

USA pin in red, clear, and blue rhinestones. Unmarked. 1940s.

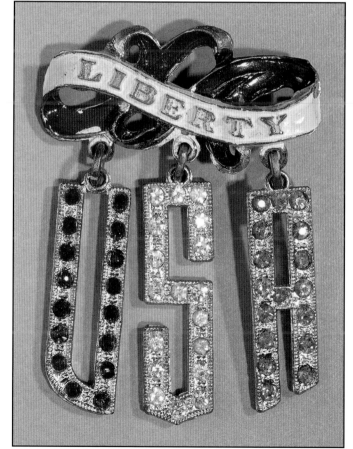

Liberty pin with dangling USA letters. Sesque-centennial, 1926. Signed by Polcini.

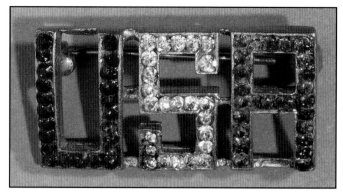

USA pin with red, clear, and blue rhinestones. Unmarked. 1940s.

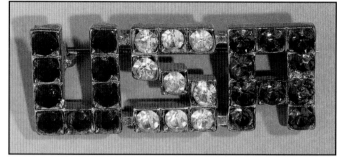

USA pin in red, clear, and blue rhinestones. Marked "Made in USA".

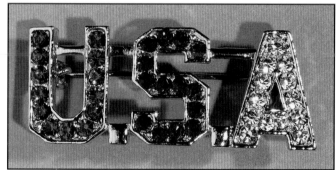

USA pin with blue, red, and clear rhinestones. Unmarked. Contemporary.

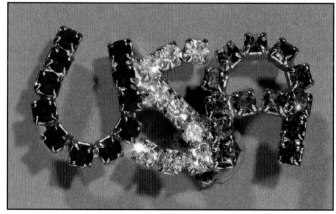

USA pin with red, clear, and blue rhinestones. Unsigned. Contemporary.

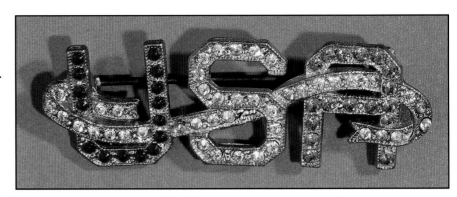

USA pin in red, clear, and blue rhinestones. Unmarked. 1940s.

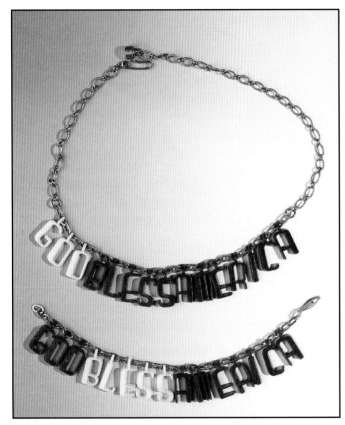

"God Bless America" necklace and bracelet in red, white, and blue plastic. 1940s.

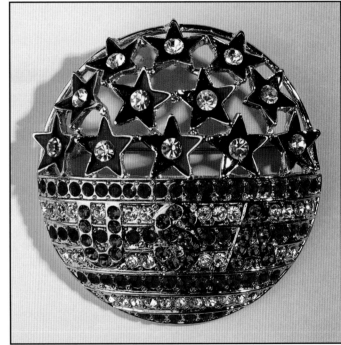

Pin with stars on top and stripes below with USA. 2 1/2" in diameter. Contemporary.

God Bless America pin with red, clear, and blue rhinestones. Contemporary.

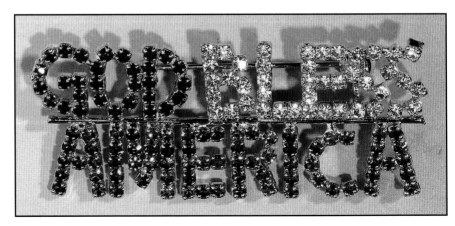

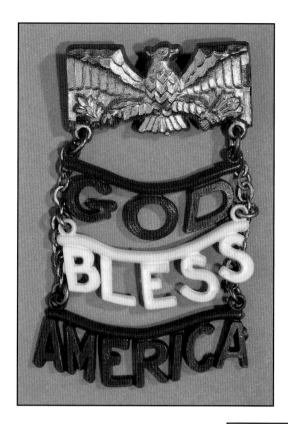

Plastic gold eagle pin with "God Bless America" in red, white, and blue letters. 1940s.

Pin reading "Frank Baby" in red, clear, and blue rhinestones. Made by Dorothy Bauer for my Dad, Frank Whitson.

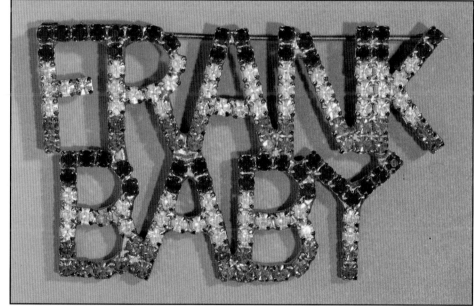

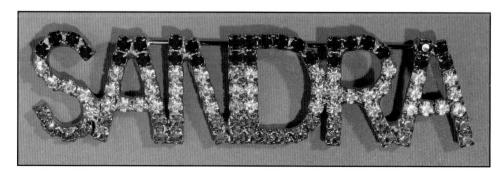

Pin that reads "Sandra" in red, clear, and blue rhinestones, made by Dorothy Bauer for me!

Show Your Colors

An eclectic group of items—in red, white, and blue colors—visually proclaim American patriotism.

Clip earrings with red, clear, and blue rhinestones. Unmarked. 1950s.

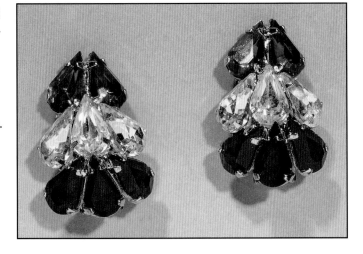

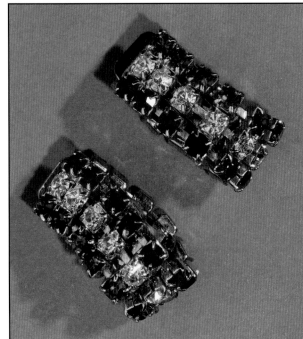

Clip earrings with red, clear, and blue rhinestones. 1950s.

2 pair square earrings with red, clear, and blue rhinestones. Unsigned. 1960s.

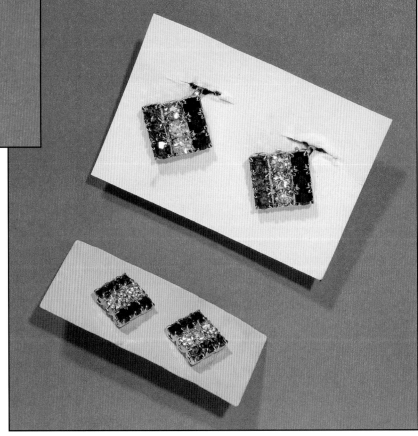

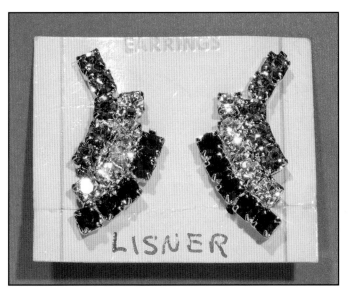

Earrings with red, clear, and blue rhinestones. By Lisner. 1950s.

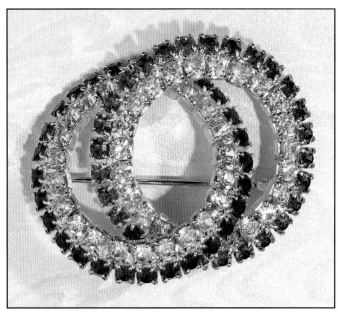

Double circle pin with red and clear, and blue and clear rhinestones. Unsigned. 1960s.

Pair of bar pins with red, clear, and blue rhinestones. Contemporary.

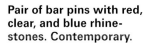

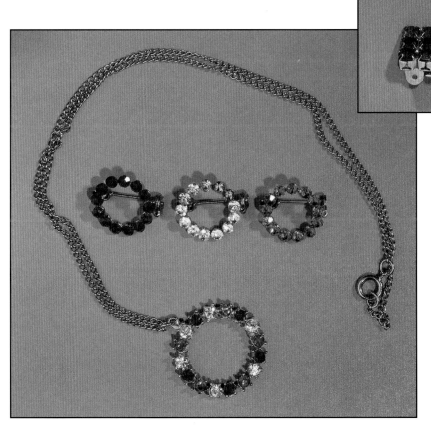

Necklace with a red, clear, and blue rhinestone pendant. Three circle scatter pins in red, and white, and blue rhinestones. Unsigned. 1960s.

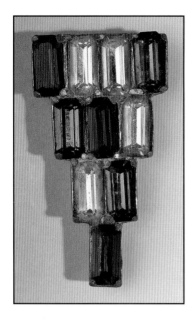

Pin with red, clear, and blue rhinestones. Courtesy of Barbara Trujillo.

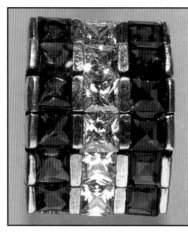

Ring with red, clear, and blue rhinestones. Courtesy of Barbara Trujillo.

Six assorted bracelets with patriotic colors. Left bracelet, 1950s. 3rd from left is marked OTC. Right bracelet, 1940s. All others contemporary.

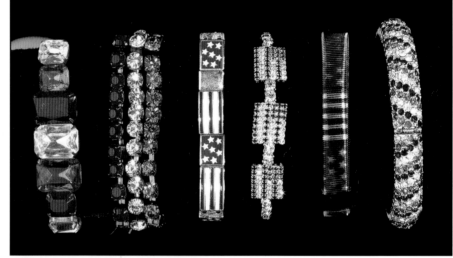

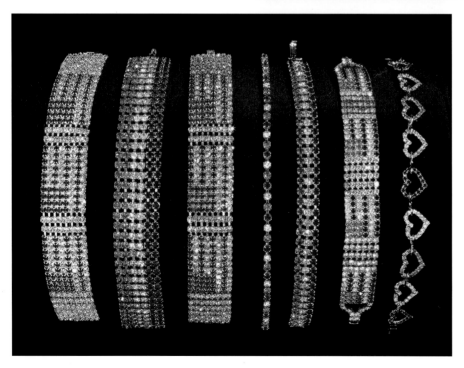

Seven assorted bracelets with patriotic colors in rhinestones. Third one from left is by Dorothy Bauer, California.

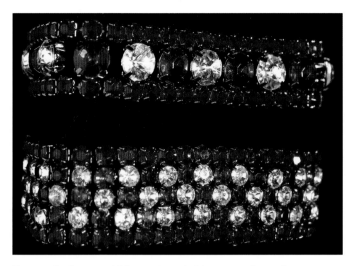

Two red, clear, and blue colored rhinestone bracelets. Contemporary.

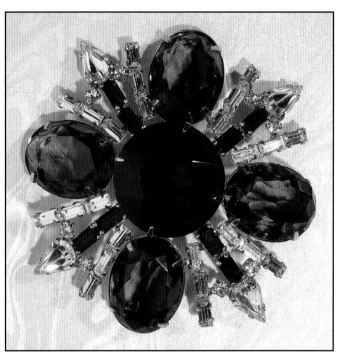

Large brooch pin with four large blue rhinestones, one large red rhinestone, and clear rhinestones. Unsigned. 1970s.

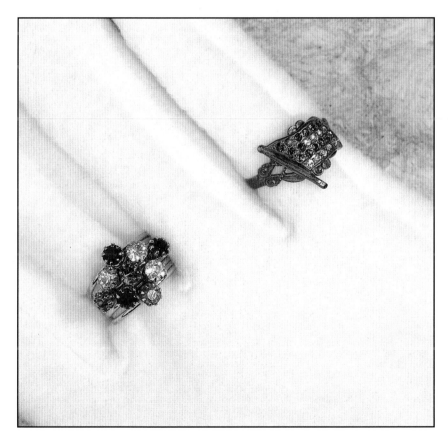

Gold ring with patriotic colored rhinestones, 1960s. Silver ring with American flag, 1940s.

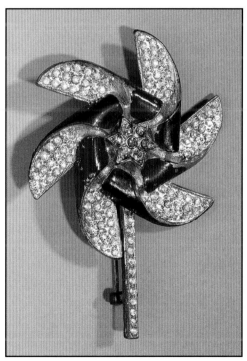

Moving pinwheel pin in red, clear, and blue rhinestones. Unmarked. 1940s.

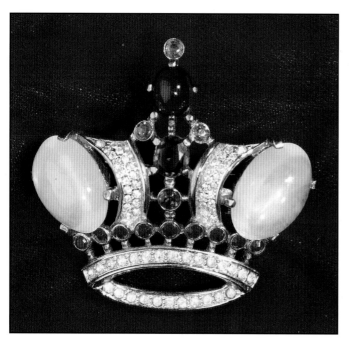

Crown pin in red, white, and blue jewels. Signed Trifari.

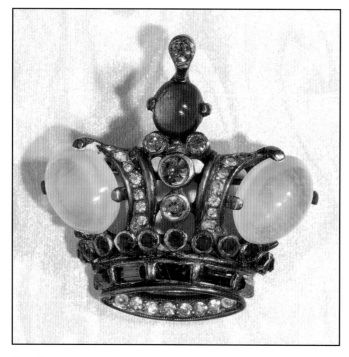

Small crown pin in red, white, and blue jewels. Signed Trifari.

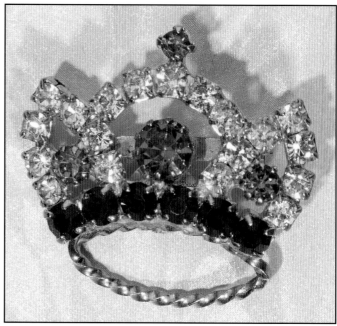

Pin in the shape of a crown with red, clear, and blue rhinestones. Unsigned. 1970s.

Two cuff links in gold with red, clear, and blue rhinestones. 1960s.

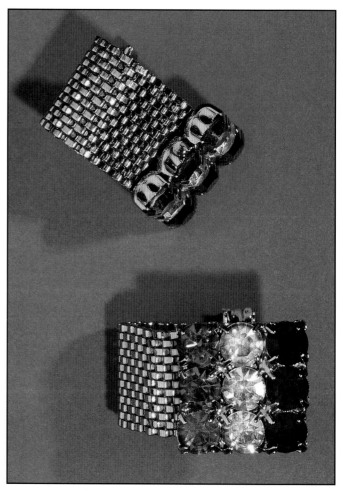

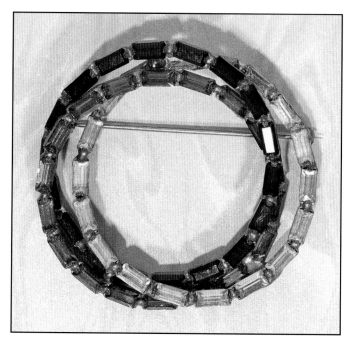

Triple Circle pin with red, clear, and blue rhinestones. Unmarked. 1940s.

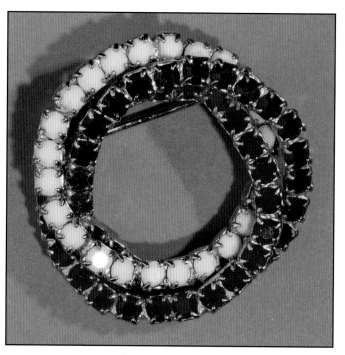

Triple circle pin in red, white milk glass, and blue opaque colors. Unsigned. 1960s.

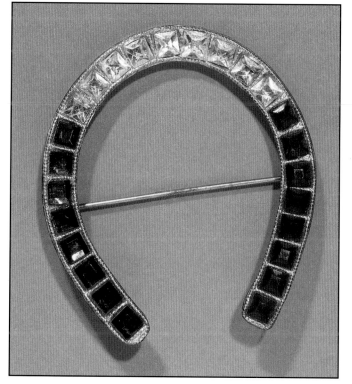

Horseshoe shaped pin with square red, clear, and blue rhinestones. Unsigned. 1940s.

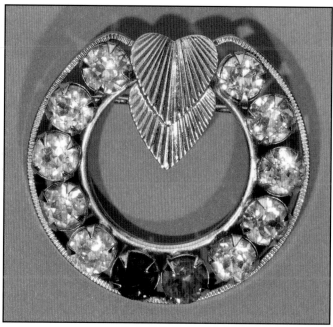

Circle pin with two hearts at the top with red, clear, and blue rhinestones. 1960s.

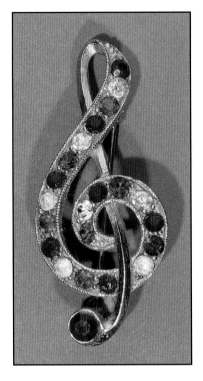

Pin in the shape of a musical note with red, clear, and blue rhinestones. Unsigned. Contemporary.

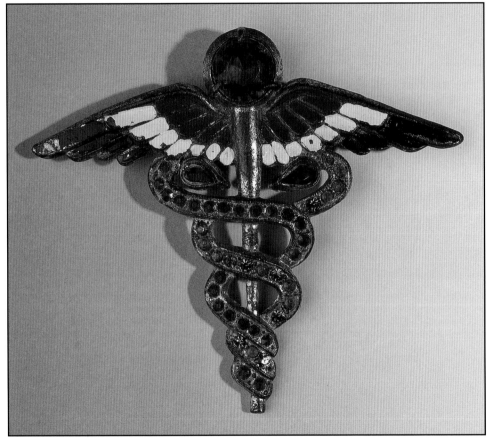

Caduceus pin with spread eagle's wings in enamel and a large blue rhinestone on top.

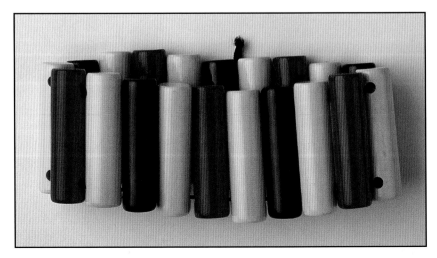

Cuff bracelet of red, white, and blue Bakelite rods between two elastic cords. 1940s.

Statue of Liberty

The Statue of Liberty was a gift to America from the people of France, in 1886. It stands in recognition of the friendship established between the two countries during the American Revolution. Sculpted by Frederic Auguste Bartholdi and titled "Liberty Enlightening the World," the statue was intended to have been completed in 1876, for the hundredth anniversary of the American Declaration of Independence. It was a joint effort, the American people were to build the pedestal and the French people were to provide the statue. Represented is a woman escaping the chains of tyranny. She holds a torch, which represents liberty, and a tablet, which is inscribed "July 4, 1776," in Roman numerals.

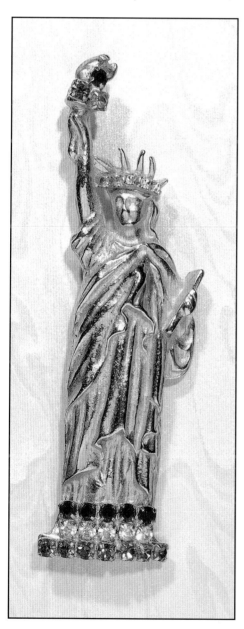

Golden Statue of Liberty pin. Signed Kirk's Folly. Contemporary.

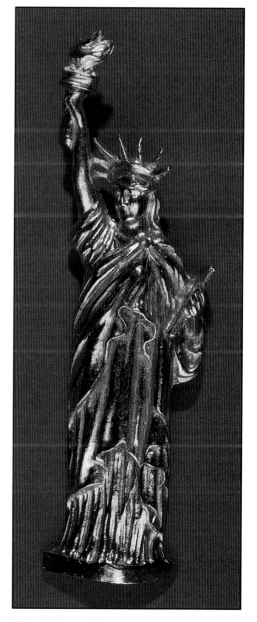

Gold Statue of Liberty pin.

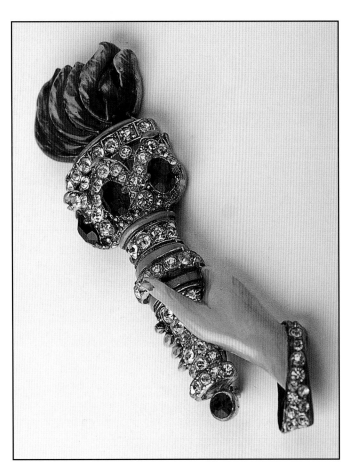

Liberty Torch pin, 1942, by Staret Jewelry Co., Inc., which was later bought out by Eisenberg. It suggests the Statue of Liberty holding a torch. 4" long. This pin was reproduced as a contemporary pin.

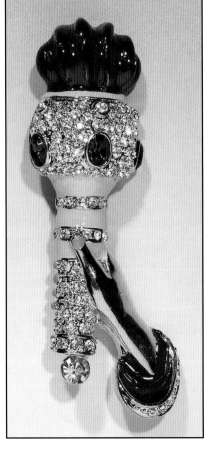

Torch pin with red, clear, and blue rhinestones. Enamel. Unsigned.

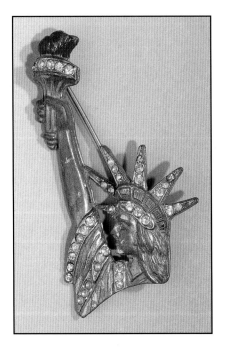

Pin with Statue of Liberty head and torch. Unsigned. 1940s.

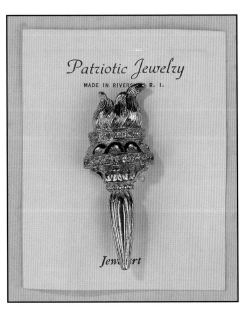

Golden torch pin. Patriotic Jewelry on original card, by Jewelart, from Riverside, R.I.

Uncle Sam

There is a debate among scholars regarding the origins of Uncle Sam. One view sites Sam Wilson, the owner of a meat packing business in Troy, New York. He supplied pork and beef to the U. S. Army during the War of 1812. The barrels of meat from his factory were first stamped "U. States," for the United States, and later the stamp read simply "US." People began saying the meat was from "U.S.", Uncle Sam (Wilson). It became a common joke. Soldiers began calling themselves Uncle Sam's Army. Soon, all government property was stamped with "U.S." and was considered Uncle Sam's. Today, the term "Uncle Sam" is a conglomerate for all government property, or the entire government itself.

Another view of the origin of the term "Uncle Sam" comes from a cartoon image of Uncle Sam, which did not appear until 1830. Uncle Sam's cartoon look comes from two earlier figures in American culture: Brother Jonathan and Yankee Doodle. Both figures were used, off and on, mostly by political cartoonists, from the early 1830s to 1861.

The well-published political cartoonist, Thomas Nast, who began making political cartoons in the 1870s, gave Uncle Sam his beard.

Artist James Montgomery Flagg painted the now-famous image of Uncle Sam on an Army Recruiting poster during Worl War Two; it says boldly, "I Want You."

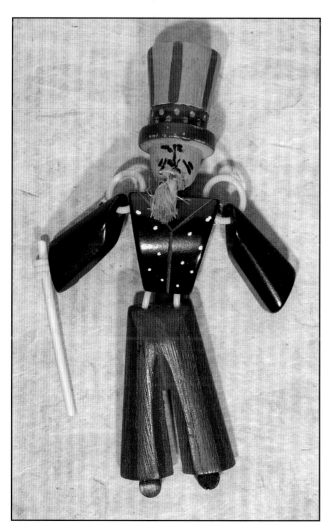

Uncle Sam pin in Bakelite and wood. 1940s.

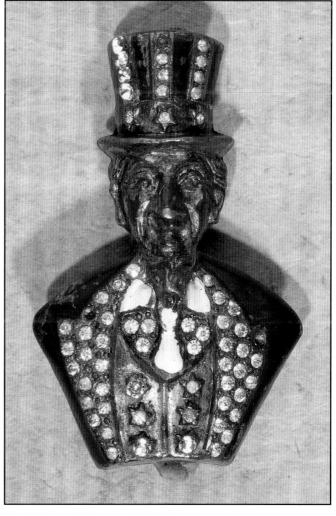

Uncle Sam pin in enamel. 1940s.

113

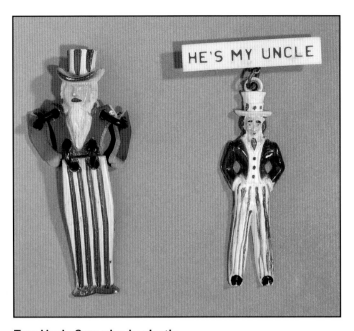

Two Uncle Sam pins in plastic.

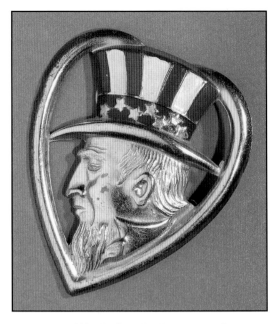

Brass pin of Uncle Sam in the center of a heart. 1940s.

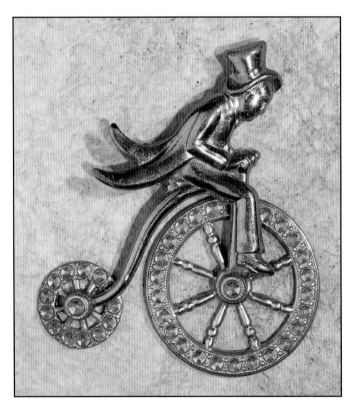

Gold pin of Uncle Sam riding a bone-cruncher bike with moving wheels. 1940s.

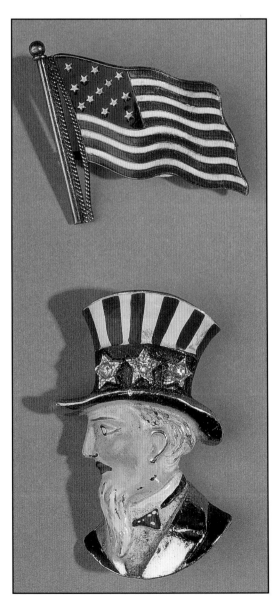

American flag pin and Uncle Sam pin.

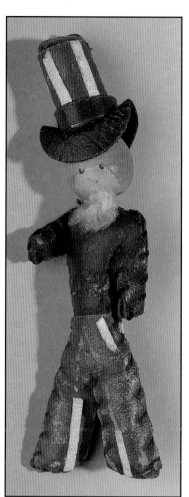

Uncle Sam pin.

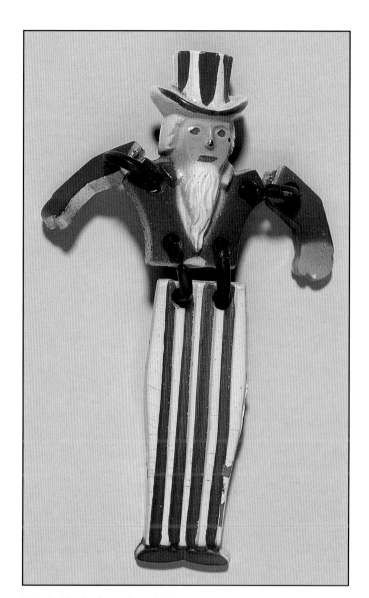

Plastic Uncle Sam pin with hinged arms and legs, painted red, white, and blue. 1940s.

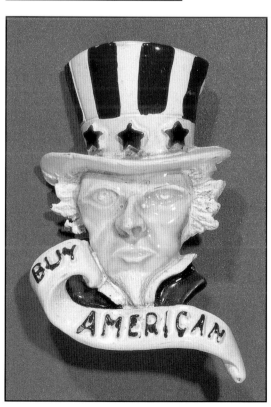

Painted metal Uncle Sam pin with banner that reads "Buy American". Contemporary.

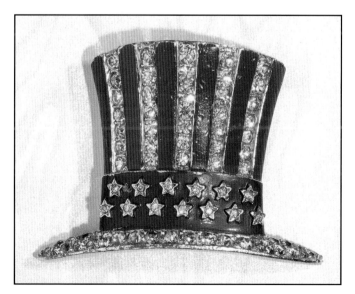

Uncle Sam hat.

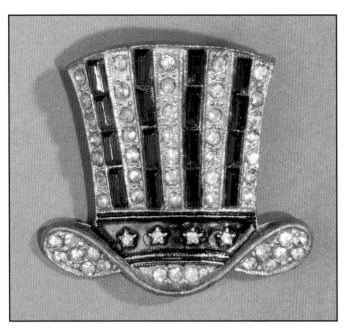

Uncle Sam hat.

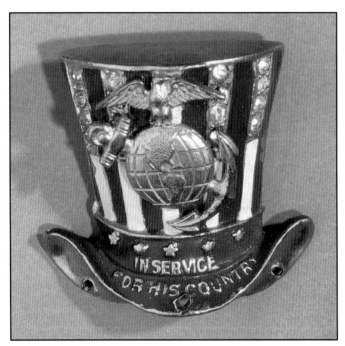

Uncle Sam hat. Enamel, missing the dangling USA letters. Solford Emblem Co.

Uncle Sam hat pin in enamel and rhinestones. Made in USA

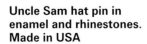

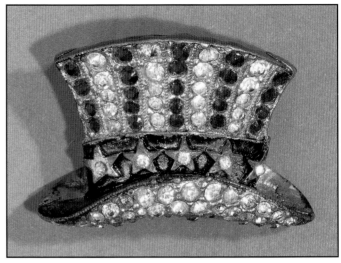

Uncle Sam hat. Unmarked. 1940s.

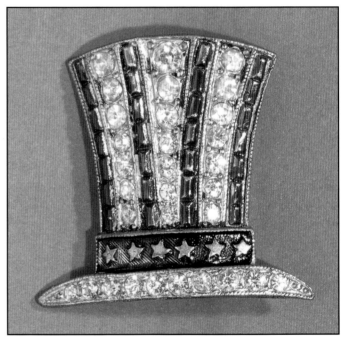

Tall Uncle Sam hat pin in rhinestones with red enamels. Unmarked. 1940s.

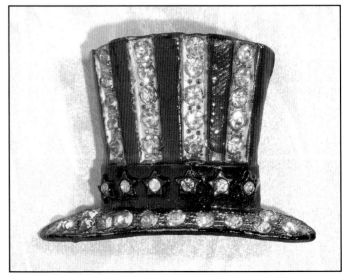

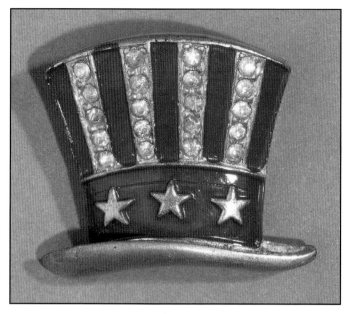

Uncle Sam hat pin in enamel. Unmarked. 1940s.

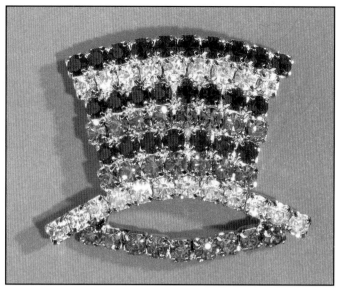

Uncle Sam hat pin, all rhinestones. 1950s-60s.

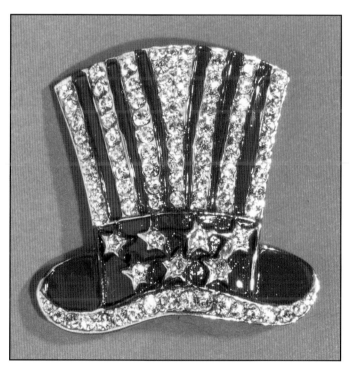

Uncle Sam hat pin. Marked Sterling. Roy Rover, New York.

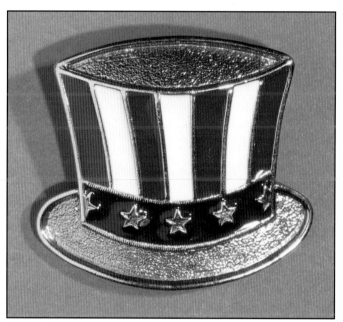

Short Uncle Sam hat pin in enamel. Unmarked. Contemporary.

Uncle Sam hat pin.
Unmarked. 1940s.

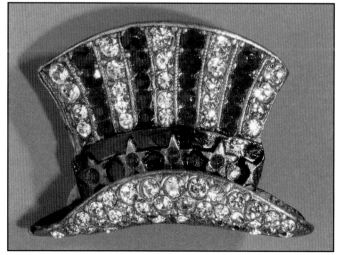

Two Uncle
Sam hat pins
in enamel and
rhinestones.

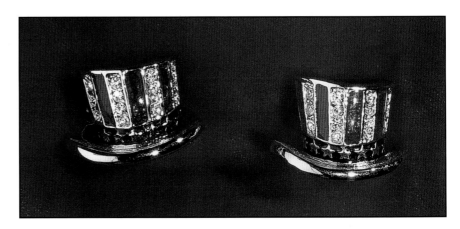

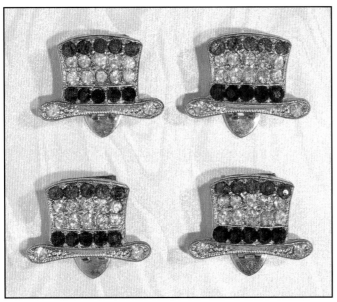

Four Uncle Sam hats in rhinestones, dress clips, unsigned.
1940s.

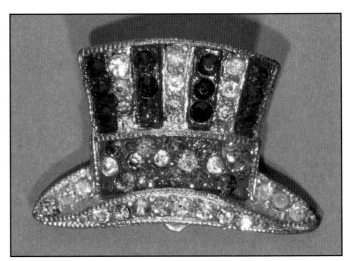

Uncle Sam hat dress clip. Unsigned. 1940s.

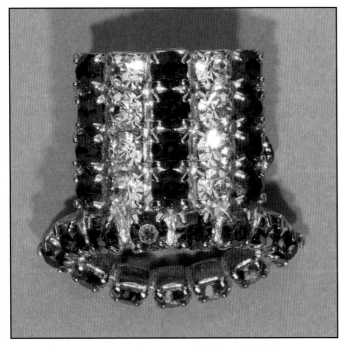

Uncle Sam hat pin in rhinestones. Unsigned. 1960s.

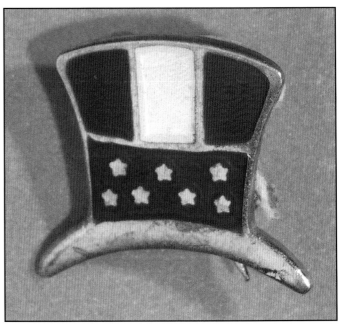

Tiny Uncle Sam hat, enamel, marked Sterling.

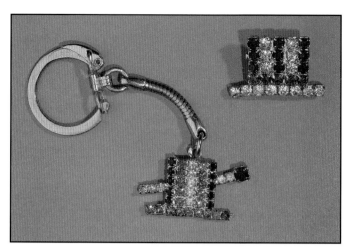

Key chain with Uncle Sam hat and Uncle Sam hat pin. Unsigned. 1960s.

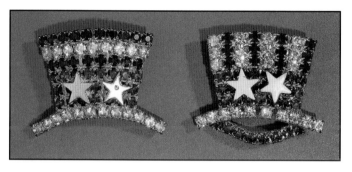

Two Uncle Sam hat pins. Unsigned. 1960s.

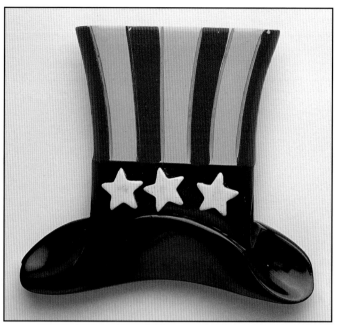

Large Bakelite top hat pin with red and white striped crown and three white stars on the dark blue hatband and brim, 2 1/4" high.

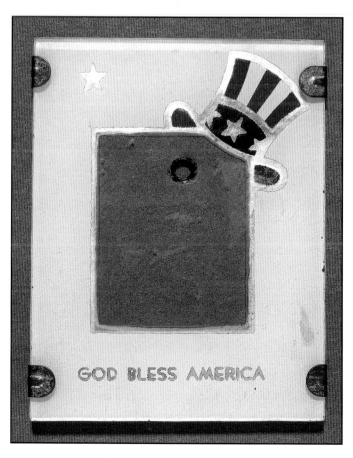

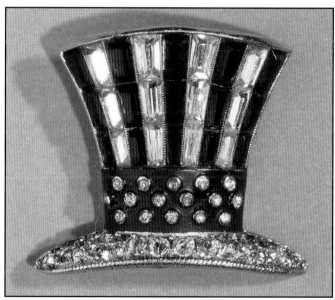

Pin of Uncle Sam hat.

Picture frame of painted glass with a stiff paper backing, marked "God Bless America." 1960s.

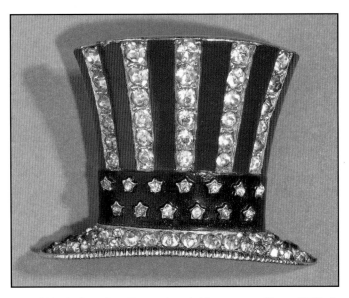

Pin of Uncle Sam hat. Enamel and rhinestones. Signed Trifari.

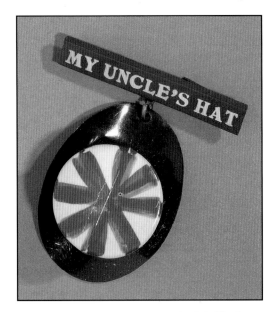

Celluloid pin that reads "My Uncle's Hat". 1940s.

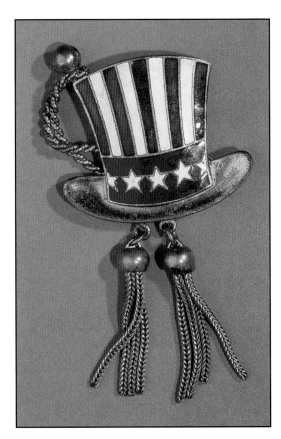

Uncle Sam hat with dangling tassels. Unsigned. 1940s.

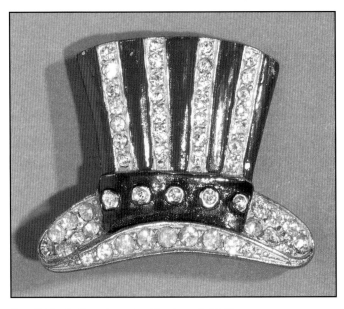

Small Uncle Sam hat pin. Unsigned. 1940s.

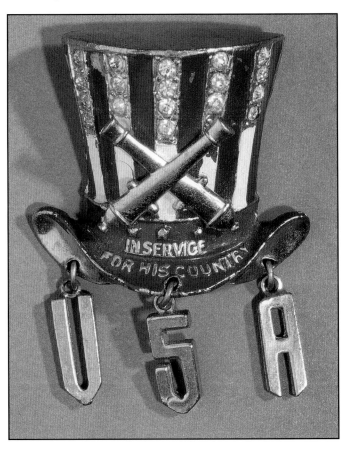

Uncle Sam hat with USA pendants. Marked FORD Emblem Co. Front marked "In Service for his Country". 1940s.

People

While World War Two raged on, many of those Americans who had loved ones in the military service wanted to show their patriotism and support. They wore many types of patriotic pins, including those showing soldiers and sailors, to honor people in different branches of military service. You will find a wide variety here.

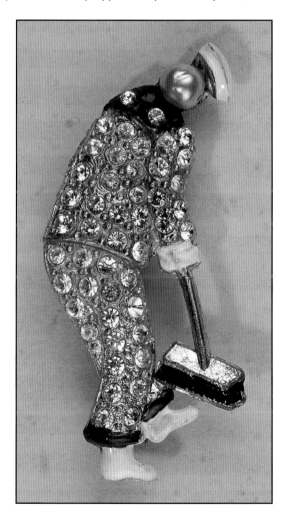

Pin of sailor man swabbing the deck. Rhinestones, enamel, and pearl. WWII period.

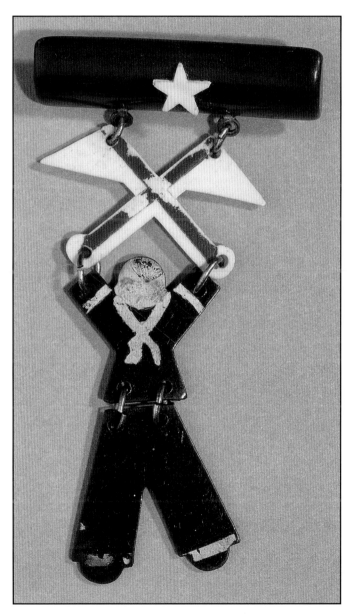

Navy pin. Dangling celluloid. 1930s.

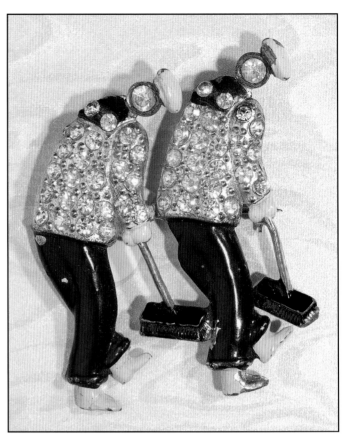

Pin of two sailors pushing brooms, rhinestones and white and blue enamel. Unmarked. 1940s.

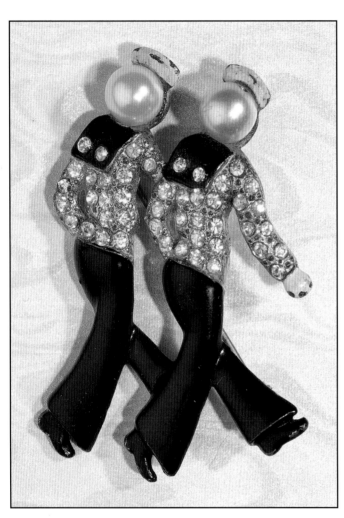

Pin of two walking sailors with white and black enamel, clear rhinestones, and pearls.

Pin with two walking sailors with white, black and blue enamel. Unmarked. 1940s.

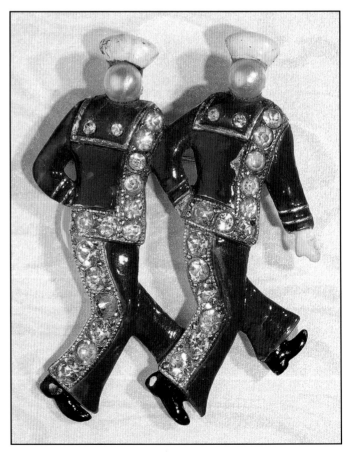

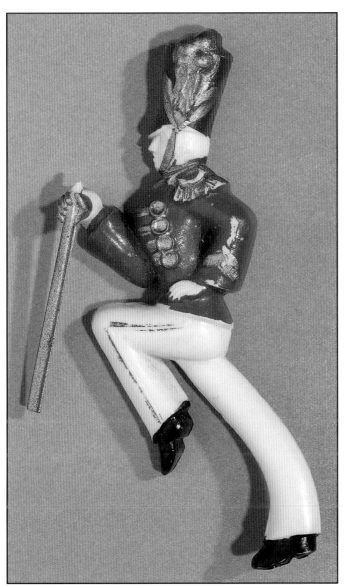

Marching majorette pin of
enameled celluloid.

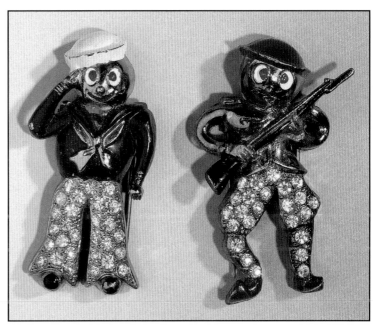

Two soldiers in black face, dress clips, marked L-N. 1940s.

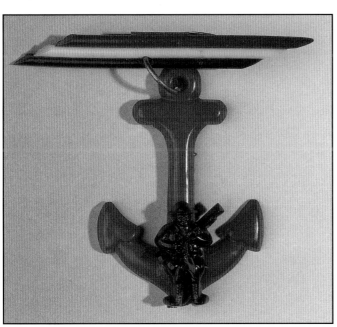

Pin with red anchor and
soldier sitting atop.

Politics

Political cartoonist Thomas Nast, who is credited with drawing the Uncle Sam figure we most recognize today, has a few more claims to fame. He designed the now-famous image of the Democratic party's mascot donkey, which was first associated with President Andrew Jackson's 1828 Presidential campaign. Jackson's opponents called him a "jackass" (donkey), and Jackson decided to use this image of the strong-willed donkey on his campaign posters. Later, Thomas Nast used the Democratic party's donkey in newspaper cartoons and made the symbol famous.

In a cartoon that appeared in Harper's Weekly in 1874, Nast drew a donkey in a lion's skin, scaring away all the animals at the zoo. One of those animals, the elephant, was labeled "The Republican Vote." From then on, the elephant became associated with the Republican party. This group includes not only donkeys and elephants, but also particular candidates' names on political pins.

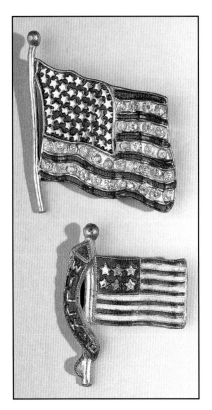

Two American flag pins, one lettered "Willkie". 1940s. Courtesy of Barbara Trujillo.

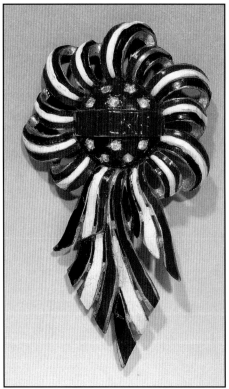

Political ribbon pin in patriotic red, white, and blue with clear rhinestones in the center. Marked "Willkie". 1940s.

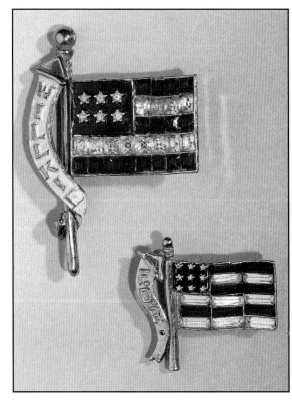

Two political American flag pins with banners on the flag poles. Unmarked. WILLKIE FDR. 1940s.

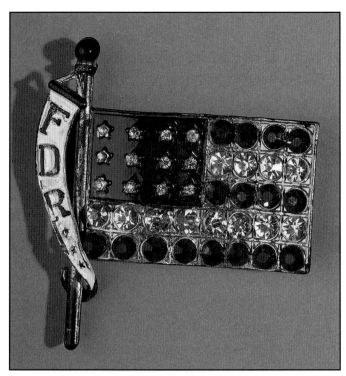

American flag with white banner reading "FDR". Unsigned. 1940s.

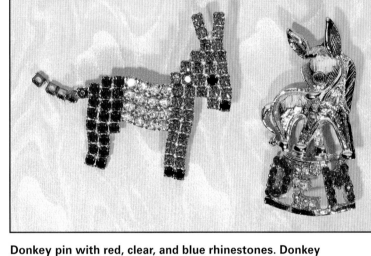

Donkey pin with red, clear, and blue rhinestones. Donkey pin with DEM(ocrat) in rhinestones. 1950.

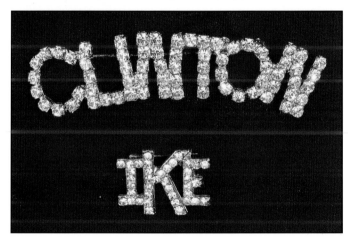

Two clear rhinestone presidential pins, "Clinton" 1990s and "Ike" 1950s. Both unsigned.

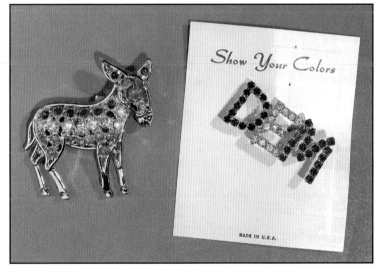

Gold donkey pin with red, clear, and blue rhinestones. DEM(ocrat) pin in red, clear, and blue rhinestones. 1960s.

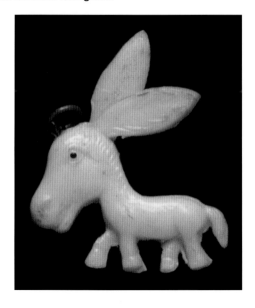

White celluloid charm of a donkey with enlarged head and black dot eye, with metal hanging ring. 1940s.

Two small gold donkey pins. 1960s.

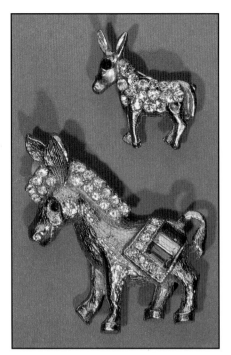

Donkey pin in pavé Aurora rhinestones and red stone eye. Original paper card with it reads, "Jewels by Cinerama, Cranston, R.I." 1950s.

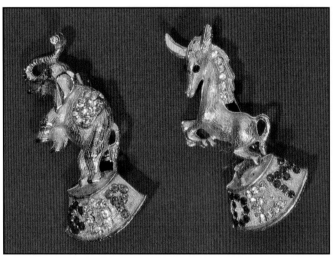

Two gold pins, one with elephant "GOP" (Grand Old Party), and one with donkey "DEM" (Democrat). 1960s.

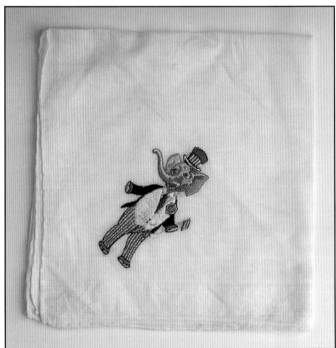

White linen handkerchief with an embroidered decoration of a standing elephant in top hat, tails coat, and striped trousers waving a red and white striped flag. 1940s.

Two silver elephant pins in red, clear, and blue rhinestones. Contemporary.

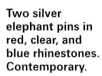

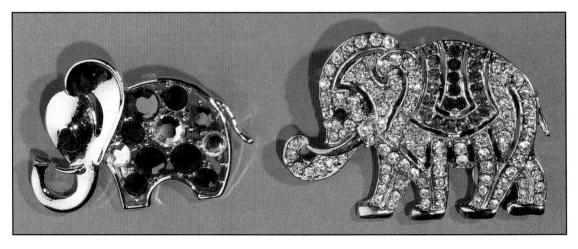

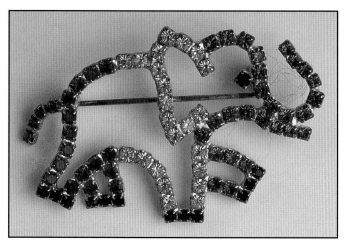

Silver metal outline of an elephant with red, white, and blue rhinestones, black eye and feet, and a flexible red tail. Contemporary.

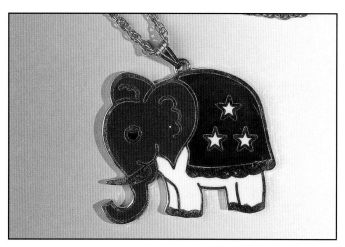

Enameled red, white, and blue elephant charm on a gold necklace. Contemporary.

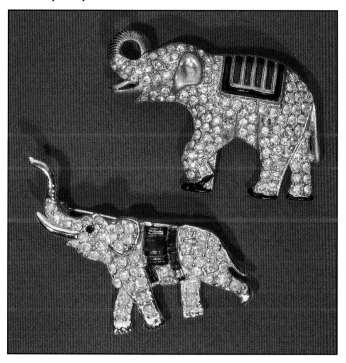

Two elephant pins with enamel and rhinestones. Top, 1940s. Bottom, 1960s.

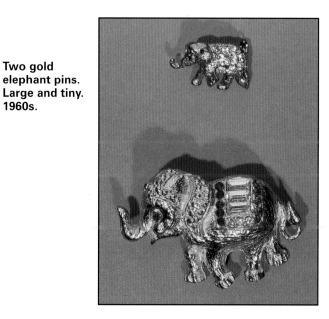

Two gold elephant pins. Large and tiny. 1960s.

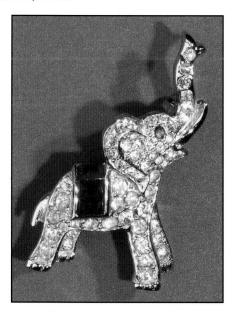

Tiny elephant pin with red blanket and green eye. Marked Pat. Pend.

Leather elephant with GOP (Grand Old Party) initials. Courtesy of Barbara Trujillo.

Airplanes

Airplanes played a strategic role in both the first and the second world wars, and patriotic airplane pins were very popular at those times. "Keep 'Em Flying" was the sentiment and a popular slogan of the day.

Silver airplane pin with red, clear, and blue rhinestones. Unmarked. 1940s.

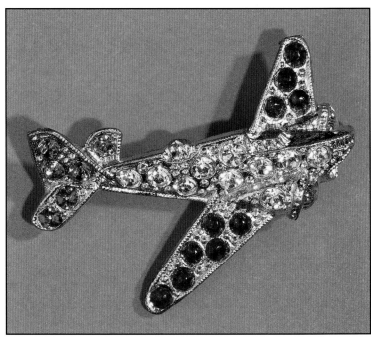

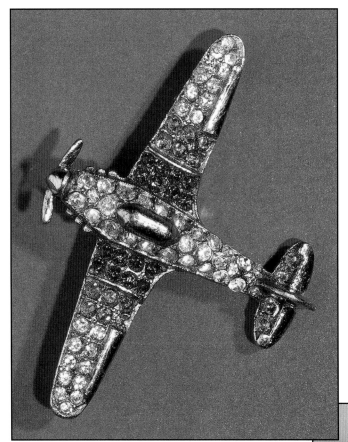

Airplane pin in silver and rhinestones.

Golden metal jet plane pin, with red, white, and blue enameled stripes and clear rhinestones. Contemporary.

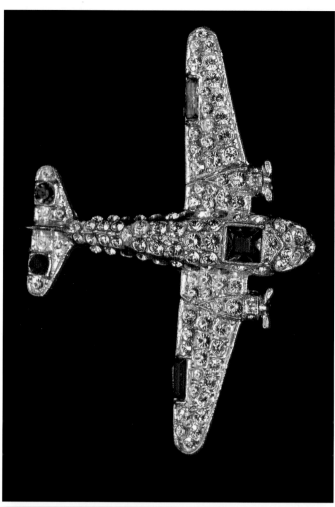

Cast pot metal propeller airplane pin with pavé rhinestones, red stone "lights" on the left side, green stone "lights" on the right side, and blue stone cockpit. Unmarked. 1940s.

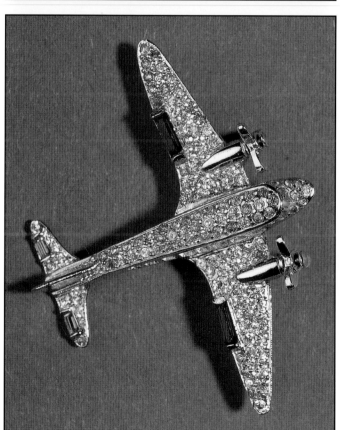

Silver pin-pendant designed as a propeller airplane with rhinestone accents and red, white, and blue baguettes in the belly. Marked "Sterling." 1940s.

Cast pot metal airplane pin with turning propellers, pavé rhinestones and red and blue "lights." Marked "Coro." Late 1940s.

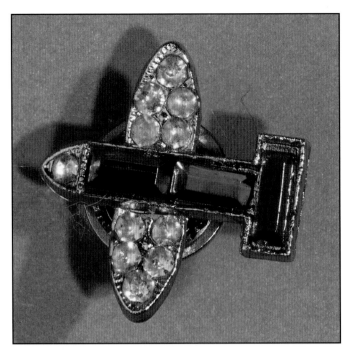

Tiny gold airplane pin with red, clear, and blue rhinestones. 1940s.

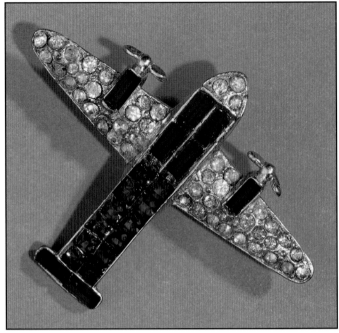

Red, white, and blue rhinestone airplane pin. Unmarked. 1940s.

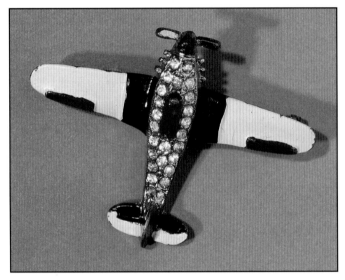

Red, white, and blue enameled airplane with clear rhinestones. Unmarked. 1940.

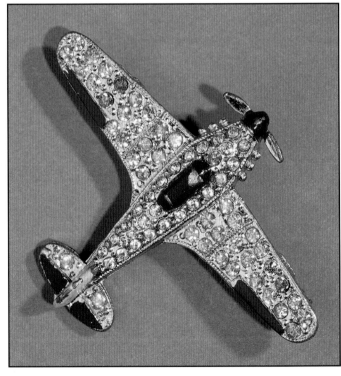

Gold airplane pin with red and clear rhinestones. Unmarked. 1940s.

Military Insignia

"Sweetheart jewelry" is a term that has come to include jewelry specifically designed to honor civilians during a time of national war. "Mother's pins," for example, were worn by a mother of someone in the military service. They signified, with a number of stars, how many children she had in the military service. There were pins that read, in script, "sweetheart," "sister," "brother," and "mother" with the same intent.

Another category in this group is images of military headgear, including a military officer's dress cap. Most of the military hat jewelry are pins that represent US Army hats; since the Army is the oldest and largest of the US Armed Forces. Other military items represented include drums, bugles, and cannons.

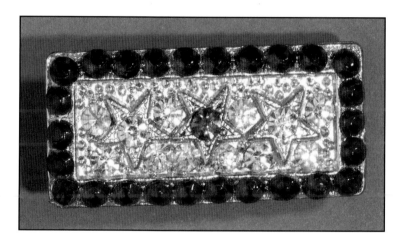

Pin with red, clear, and one blue rhinestone. Mother pins with number of sons in service.

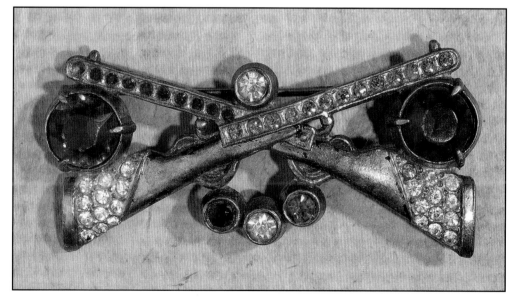

Pin with red, clear, and blue rhinestones. Unmarked. 1940s.

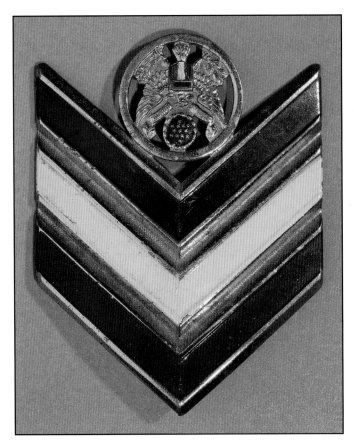

Pin with brass eagle on top and triple V, in red, white, and blue colors.

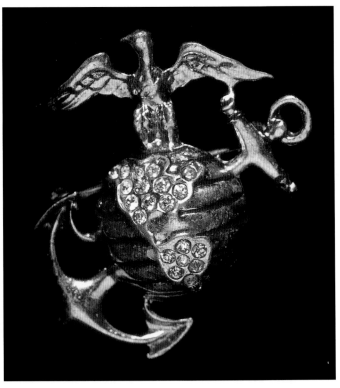

Pin of stamped metal and the eagle, anchor, and globe insignia of U. S. Marines, traces of red enamel, marked Sterling. 1940s.

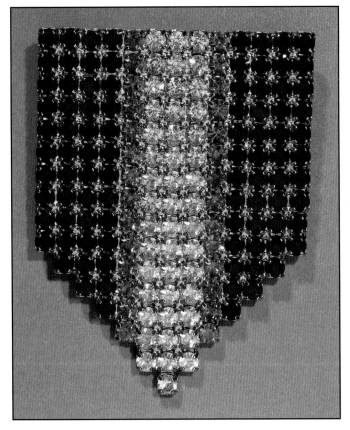

Pin with red, clear, and blue rhinestones. Signed by Dorothy Bauer.

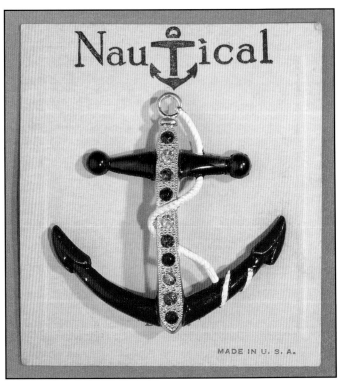

Nautical anchor pin in red, white, and blue colors on card. Enamel and rhinestones.

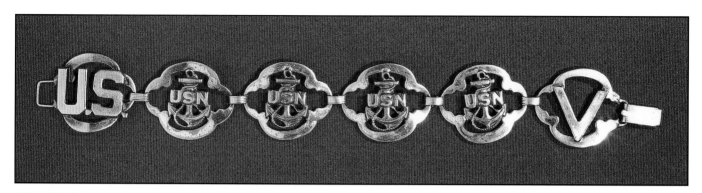

Silver link bracelet with US, USN, and V links. Marked Sterling. 1940s.

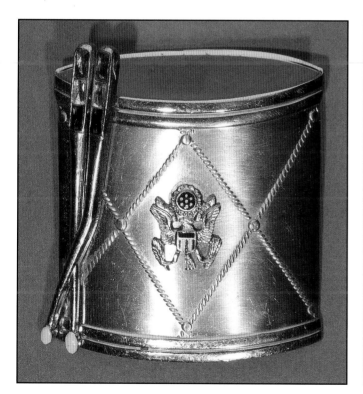

Silver drum and drumsticks with crest on front. Marked. ©
RA. 1940s.

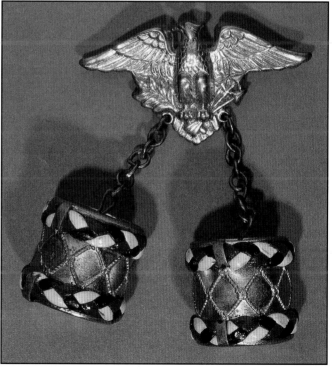

Gold eagle with two dangling drum ornaments. Unmarked.
1940s.

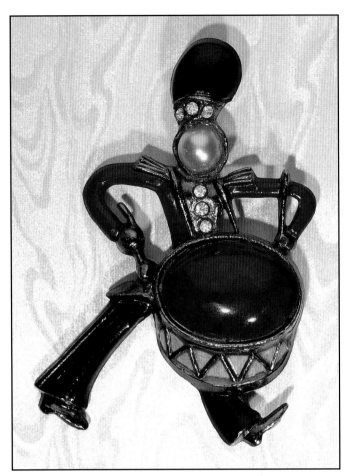

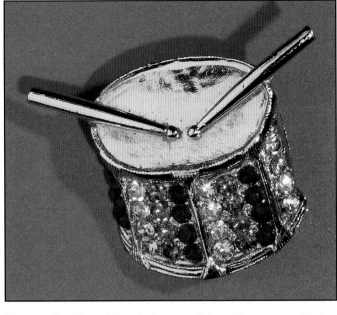

Drum and sticks with red, clear, and blue rhinestones. 1960s.

Drummer boy playing the drum. Enamel and red cabochon. Pearl face. 1930-40s.

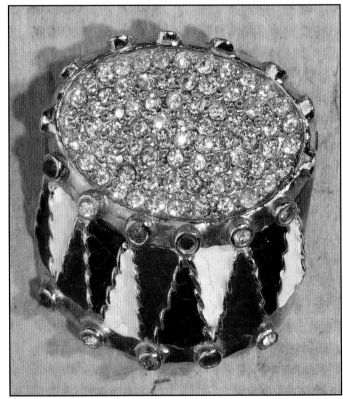

Drum pin with enameled red, clear, and blue rhinestones. Unmarked. 1950s.

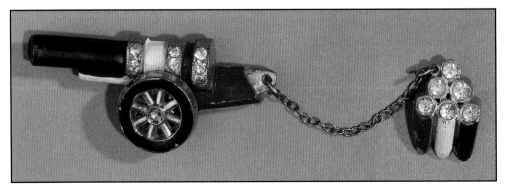

Cannon with attached cannon balls. Enamel and rhinestones.

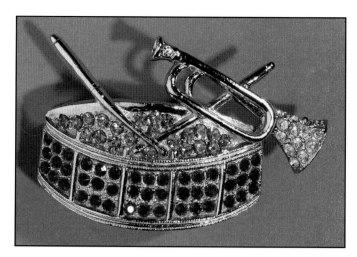

Drum with red and blue rhinestones with clear colored horn attached.

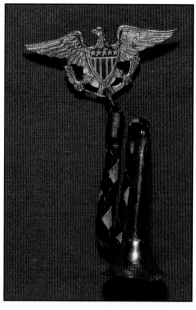

Stamped metal eagle with enameled shield insignia pin, and a pendant bugle design with woven gimp and brass horn. Unmarked. 1940s.

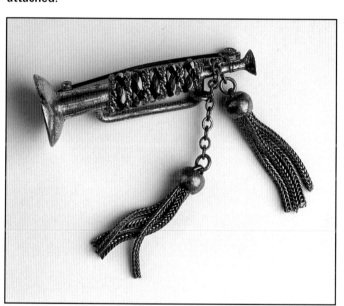

Brass bugle pin with red, white, and blue gimp and gold rope coiled around the horn and two gold tassels hanging from the mouthpiece end. 1940s.

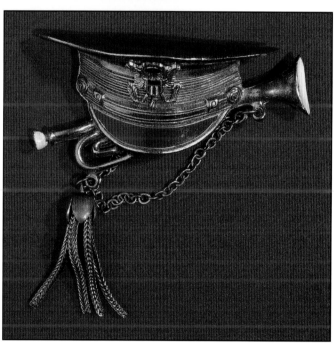

Gold soldier hat with horn and dangling tassel in metal with enamel. Patent applied for 1940s.

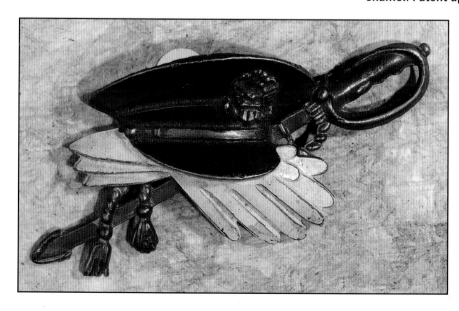

Sword pin with military emblem hat and gloves.

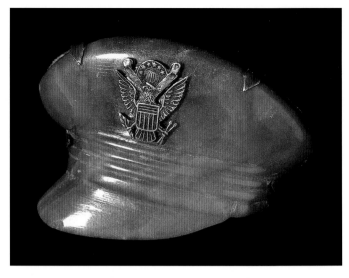

Pin in the shape of a U. S. Army cap with officer's eagle insignia, green stone and silver. Marked "Made In Mexico Sterling." 1940s.

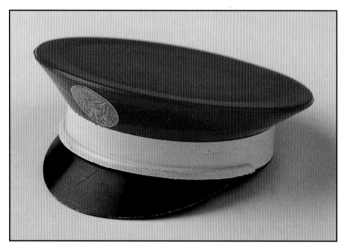

Hinged powder compact in the shape of an officer's cap, in red, white, and blue Bakelite with gold U.S. Army insignia, interior powder puff, screen, and mirror. 3" diameter. 1940s.

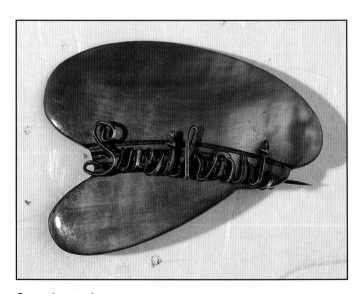

Sweetheart pin.

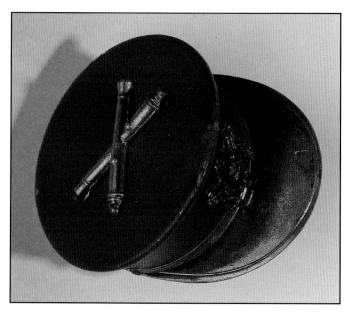

Red and gold colored soldier hat with crossed artillery cannon on top.

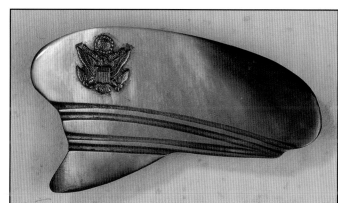

Army hat pin made of Mother of Pearl. WWII period.

Early military helmet with plume and American crest. World War II period.

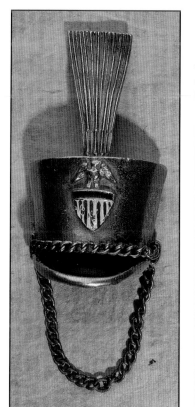

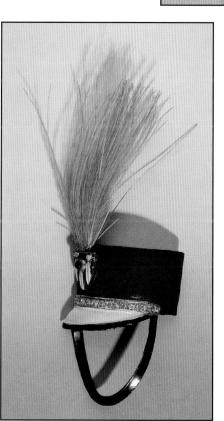

Early painted military helmet with plume and American crest pin. Rhinestone decoration. World War II period.

Hearts

Hearts are a cherished part of World War II pins and lockets. Often, the lockets open, so that a photograph of a loved one can be placed inside. How appropriate it is that these were worn on a metal chain close to the wearer's heart.

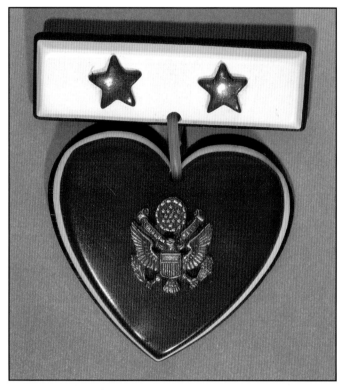

Bakelite pin with layered dangling red heart and crest in the middle. 1940s.

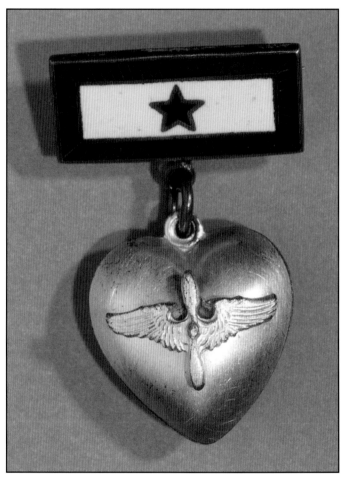

Pin with dangling silver enamel heart. Marked Sterling. A mother's pin.

Layered Bakelite pin with "Mother" on top plate with a dangling red heart. 1940s.

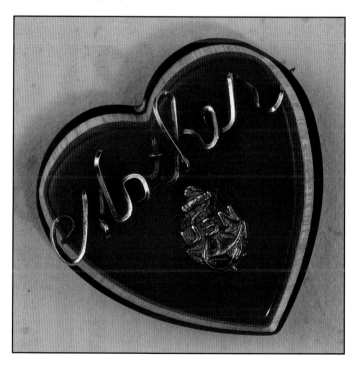

Bakelite heart pin, 3 layers of blue, white, and red. Wire letters spell "Mother" with Navy insignia.

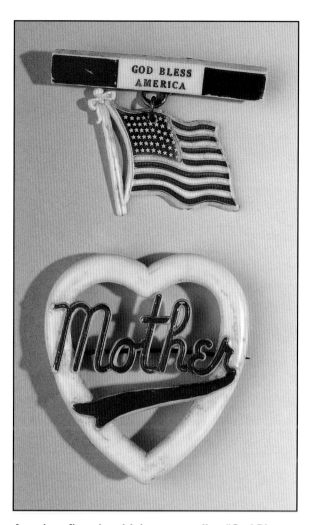

American flag pin with banner reading "God Bless America". Heart pin with "Mother" in the center. Courtesy of Barbara Trujillo.

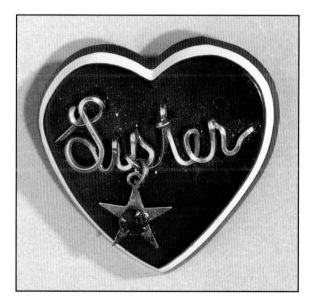

Layered Bakelite blue heart sister pin with red and white stripe and star with red rhinestone.

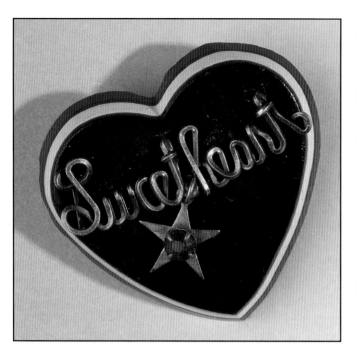

Layered Bakelite pin in the shape of a heart with "Sweetheart" and star in the center. 1940s.

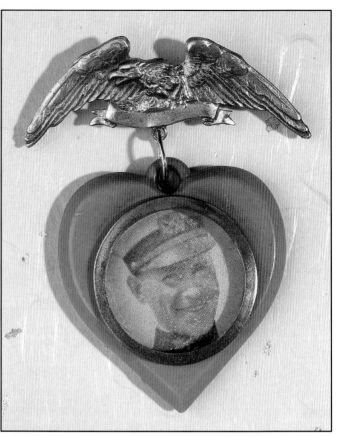

Silver eagle pin with heart photo frame. Courtesy of Barbara Trujillo.

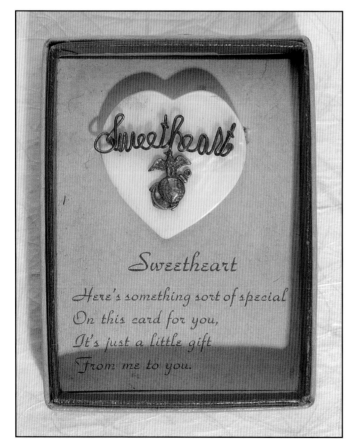

Sweetheart pin in original box with touching poem. World War II period.

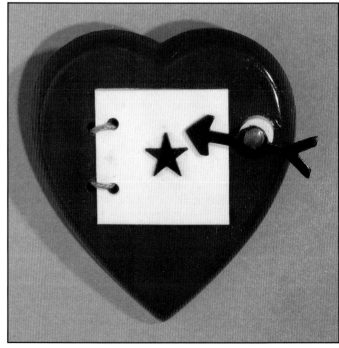

Celluloid plastic red heart pin holds a photo and is kept closed with a black arrow. 1940s.

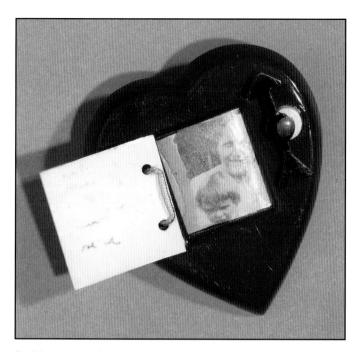

Red heart pin shown open.

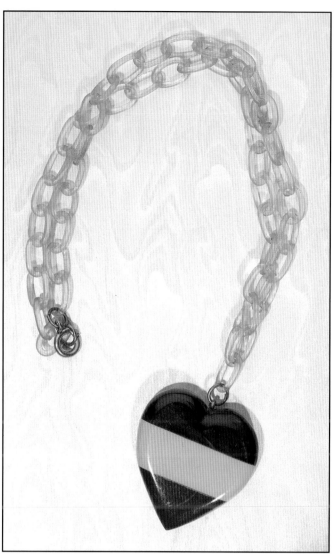

Lucite chain necklace with Bakelite heart emblem. 1940s.

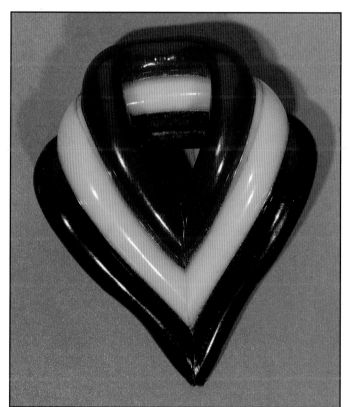

Bakelite triple heart pin in red, white, and blue. 1940s.

Gold heart pin with red, clear, and blue rhinestones representing the stripes of the flag. 1960s.

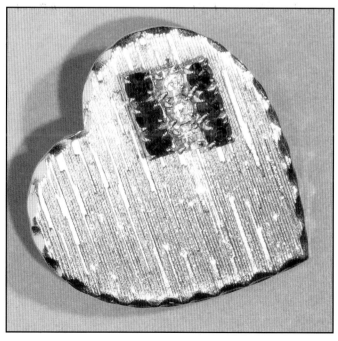

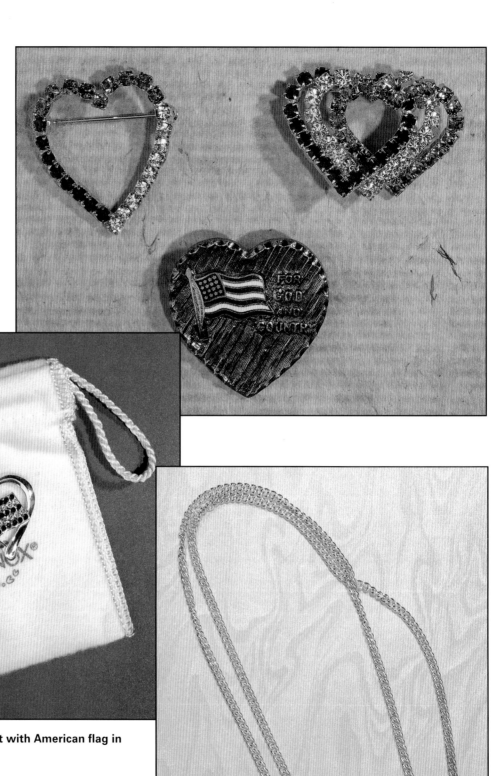

3 heart pins. "For God and Country". All un-signed. 1960s.

Silver necklace by Lenox of a heart with American flag in the center. Contemporary.

Silver chain neck-lace with heart shaped locket in red, white, and blue enamel. Unsigned. Contemporary.

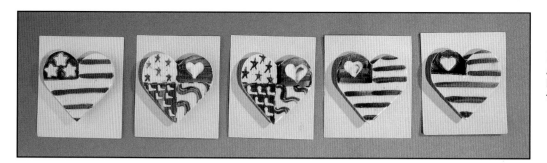

Five heart-shaped American flag ceramic button covers. Contemporary.

Patriotic pin. I Love Flag, unsigned. Enameled lapel pin, unsigned. Earrings in rhinestones by Dorothy Bauer.

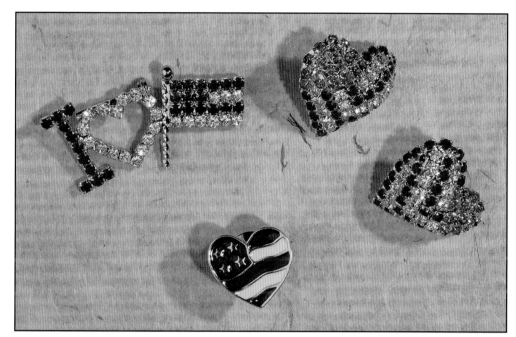

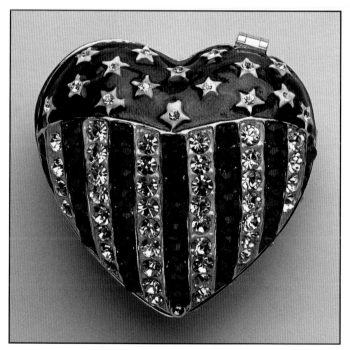

Enameled heart-shaped box with hinged lid featuring red and clear faceted rhinestone stripes and blue enamel field with white stars and "diamond" accents, 1 5/8" wide. Contemporary.

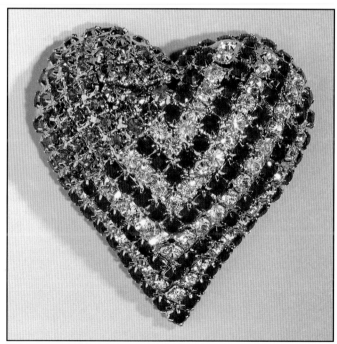

Pin in the shape of a domed heart with red, clear, and blue rhinestones, by Dorothy Bauer. 2" wide. Contemporary.

143

V for Victory

Late in the Second World War, British Prime Minister Winston Churchill raised his hand and extended his fingers to make a "V" sign to symbolize "V for Victory." In the Morse Code, three dots and a dash (. . . —) represent the letter "V." Therefore, some of the patriotic jewelry made in the 1940s incorporates both the "V" and the Morse Code symbols. Composer Ludwig van Beethoven's Fifth Symphony opens with three short notes and a long note, in the rhythm of the Morse Code "V" symbol. These became popular. The "V" symbol, in altered form, went on to become a symbol for peace during the popular movement to end the Viet Nam conflict of the 1960s. President Richard Nixon's final gesture, as he boarded an airplane after his impeachment, was to make a peace or victory sign with his hand.

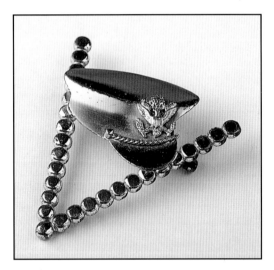

Sterling silver pin with an Army officer's cap and V for Victory, 2 1/8" high, 1940s.

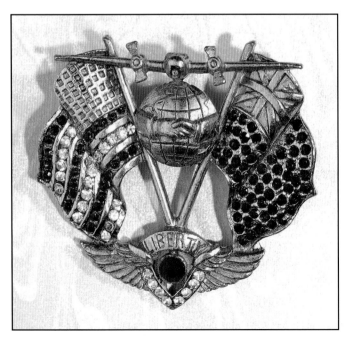

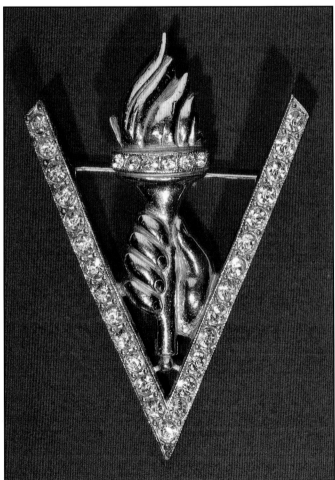

Victory V pin with gold hand holding a gold torch in the center. Unmarked. 1940s.

Gold Victory pin has waving flags and the earth shows two hands shaking. British and American insignia. Unmarked. 1940s.

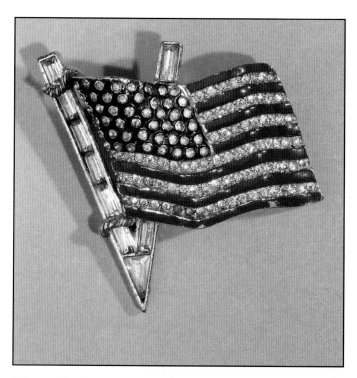

Victory pin with American flag. Enamel with baguette rhinestones, unsigned.

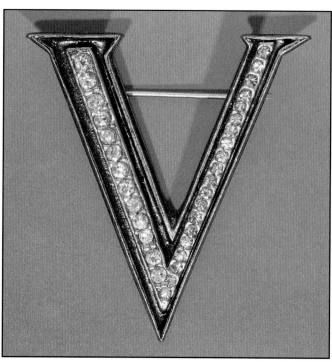

Victory pin. Unmarked. Enamel and rhinestone. 1940s.

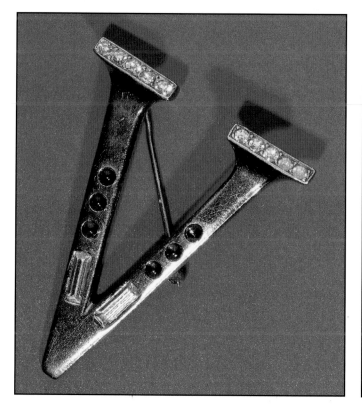

Victory pin with three dots and a dash, the Morse code signal for V. Marked Sterling. Signed Trifari. 1940s.

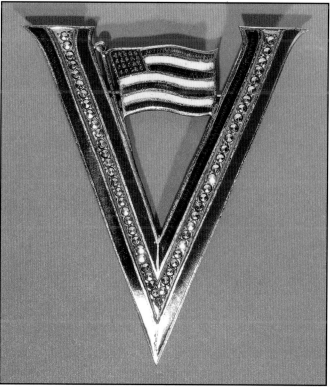

Large Victory pin with American flag in the center. Marked Sterling. 2 1/2" tall.

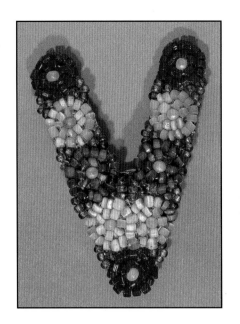

Victory pin with red, clear, and blue beads. French, 1940s.

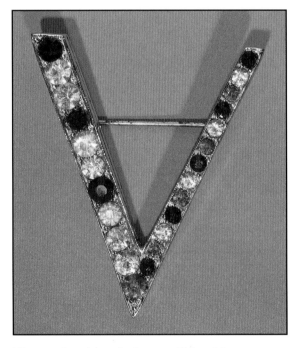

Victory pin with red, clear, and blue rhinestones. Unmarked. 1940s.

Victory pin with red, clear, and blue rhinestones. Marked Sterling. 1940s.

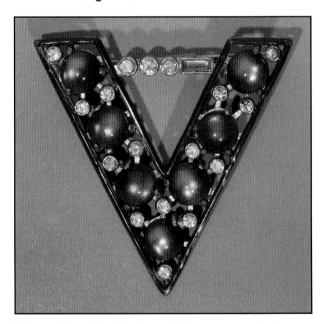

Victory pin with pink star spphire stones and clear rhinestones signifying "dot, dot, dot, dash," the Morse code letter V. Unmarked. 1940s.

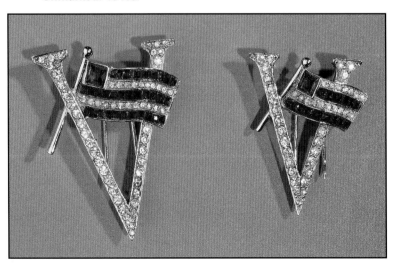

Two Victory dress clips with jeweled V American flags in the center. Unmarked. 1940s.

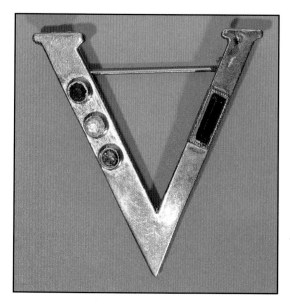

Silver Victory pin with red, clear, and blue rhinestones signifying "dot, dot, dot, dash," the Morse code letter V. Unmarked. 1940s.

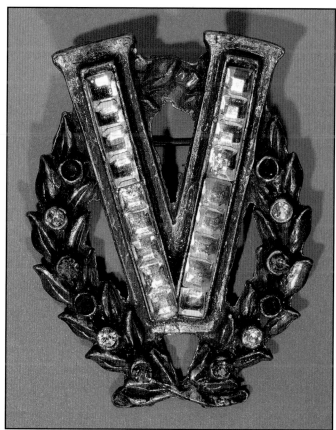

Red Victory pin in laminated Bakelite. "Mother". 1940s.

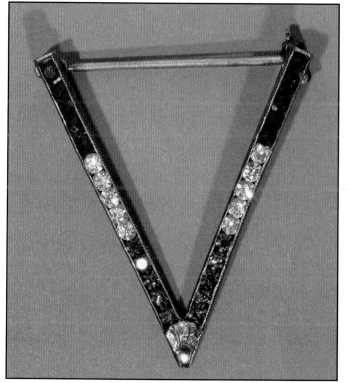

Victory pin with red, clear, and blue rhinestones. Marked Sterling.

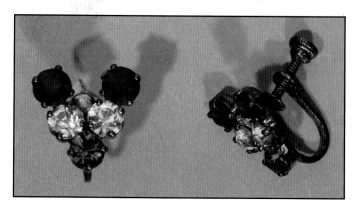

Victory pin with olive braches on either side. Unmarked. 1940s.

Pair of earrings in red, clear, and blue rhinestones. Screw-backs. 1940s.

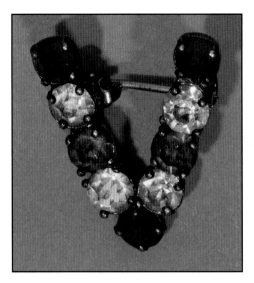

Small Victory pin with red, clear, and blue rhinestones. Marked Sterling. 1940s.

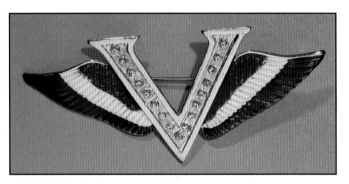

Victory pin with spread eagle's wings in red, white, and blue enamel on metal. Unmarked. Contemporary.

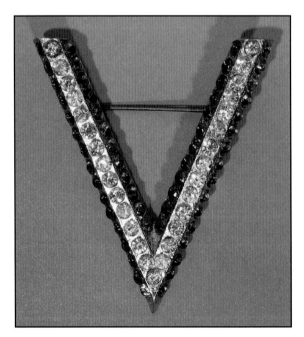

Victory pin with red, clear, and blue rhinestones on three sides. Unsigned. 1940s.

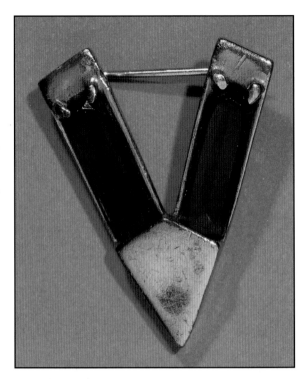

Small Victory pin. Unmarked, 1940s.

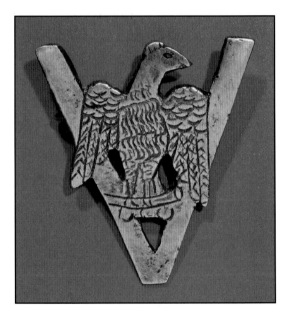

Silver Victory pin with eagle in the center. Marked 800. 1940s.

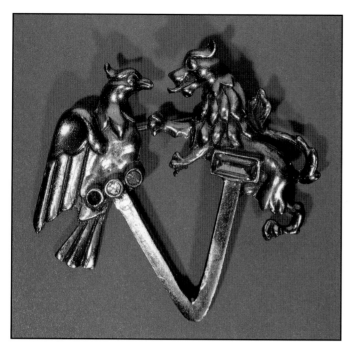

Gold Victory pin with eagle and lion on either side. Morse code. Unmarked. 1940s.

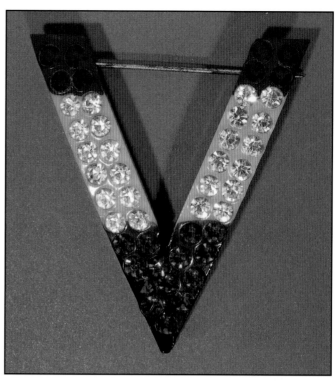

Plastic Victory pin with red, clear, and blue rhinestones. Unmarked. 1940s.

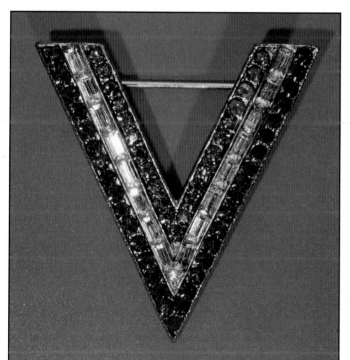

Victory pin in red, clear, and blue rhinestones. Unmarked. 1940s.

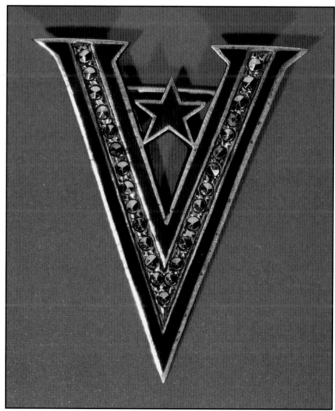

Victory pin in enamel. Marked Sterling with marcasite.

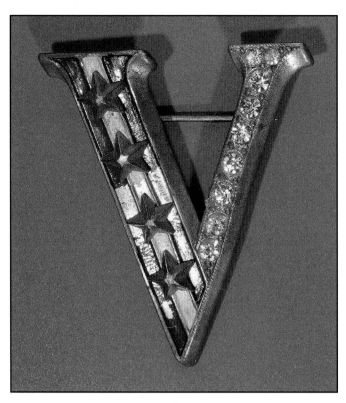

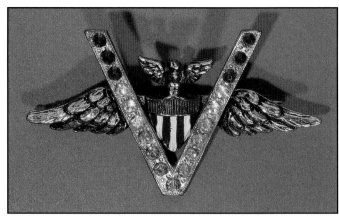

Victory pin with eagle and crest in the center and spread eagle's wings on either side. Unmarked. 1940s.

Victory pin with 4 stars on one side. Unmarked. 1940s.

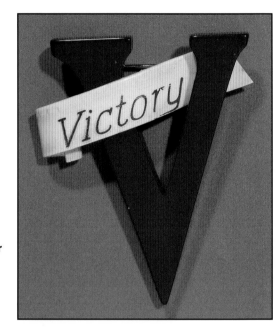

Red plastic Victory pin with white banner reading "Victory".

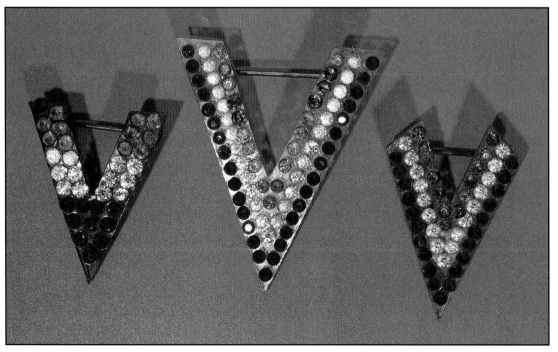

Three plastic Victory pins with red, clear, and blue rhinestones.

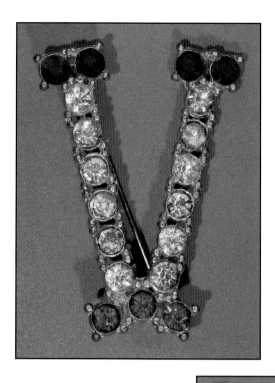

Victory pin of rhine-
stones, unmarked. 1940s.

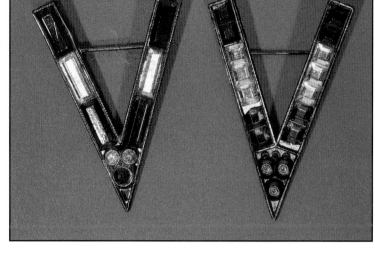

Two Victory pins with rhinestones. Unmarked. 1940s.

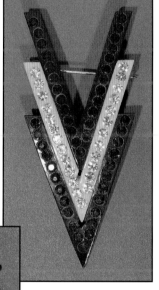

Triple line Victory
plastic pin in red,
white, and blue.

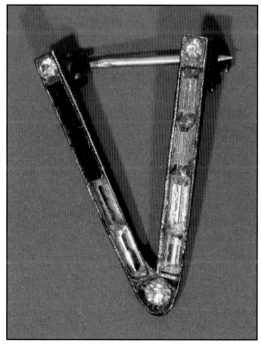

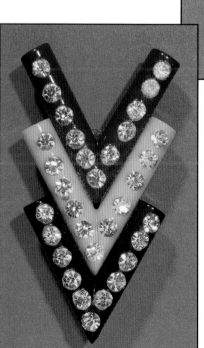

Bakelite triple
Victory pin in red,
white, and blue
with clear rhine-
stones. 1940s.

Small Victory pin with baguette rhinestones.
Unmarked. 1940.

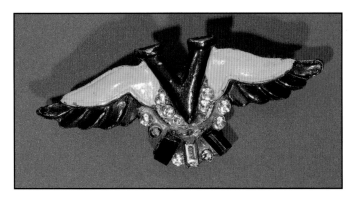

Enameled Victory pin with spread eagle's wings in red, white, and blue rhinestones. Unmarked. 1940s.

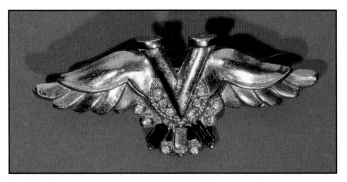

Gold Victory pin with spread eagle's wings with three baguette rhinestones.

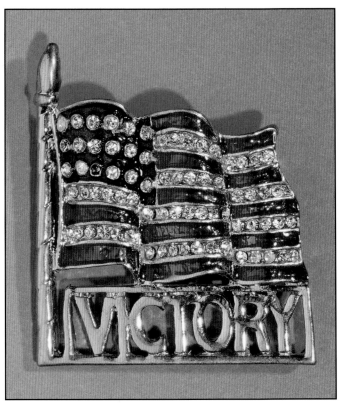

Gold waving American flag pin with "Victory" banner underneath flag. Contemporary.

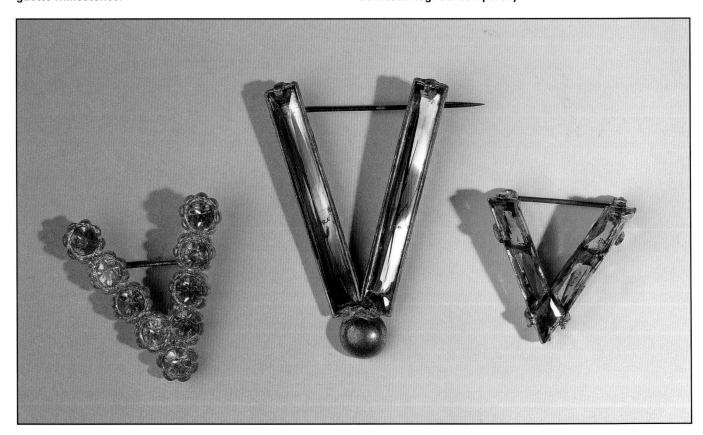

Three Victory pins. Courtesy of Barbara Trujillo.

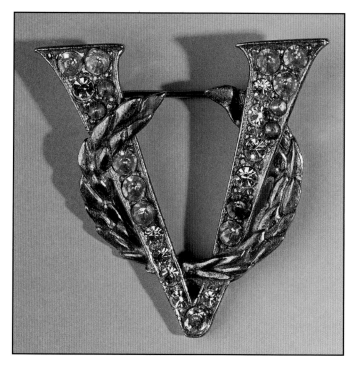

Gold Victory pin. Courtesy of Barbara Trujillo.

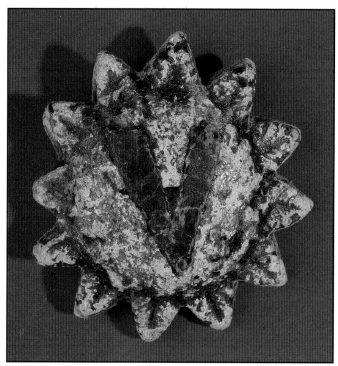

Victory pin, V on sunburst. Courtesy of Barbara Trujillo.

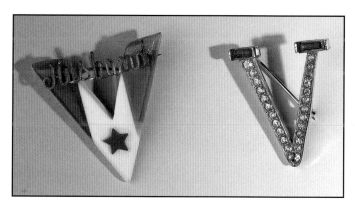

Victory pin with "Husband" on top. Victory pin in silver with two blue rhinestones on top. Courtesy of Barbara Trujillo.

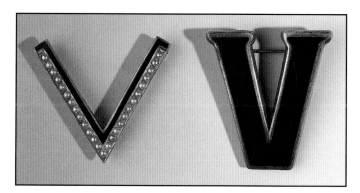

Two Victory pins. Courtesy of Barbara Trujillo.

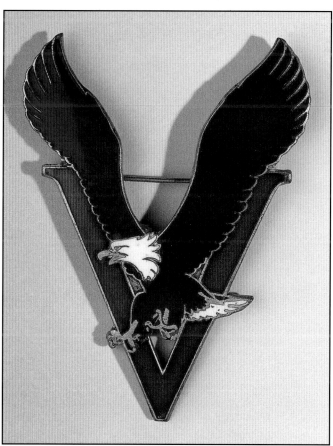

Victory pin with eagle in the center with wings spread. Courtesy of Barbara Trujillo.

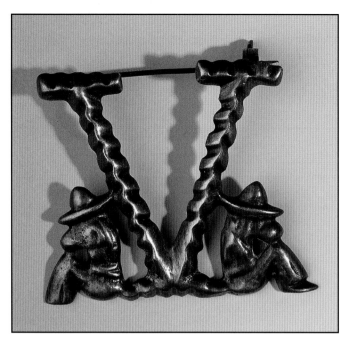

Victory pin. Courtesy of Barbara Trujillo.

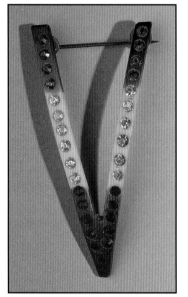

Victory pin in red, white, and blue colors and rhinestones. Courtesy of Barbara Trujillo.

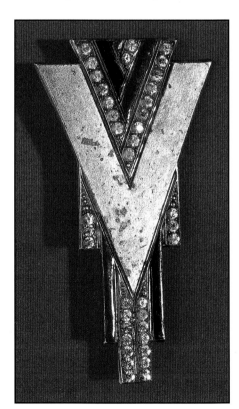

Victory pin with "Victory" on top of pin and the Morse code signal for V. Courtesy of Barbara Trujillo.

Victory pin. Courtesy of Barbara Trujillo.

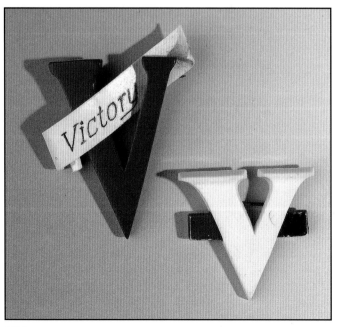

Victory pin with banner reading "Victory". Victory pin in red, white, and blue colors. Courtesy of Barbara Trujillo.

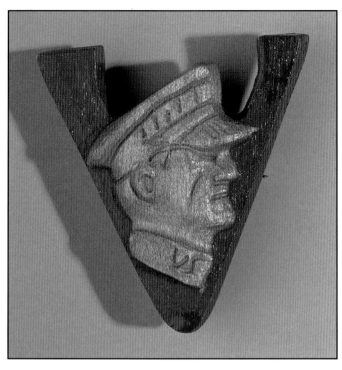

Victory pin with soldier in the middle. Courtesy of Barbara Trujillo.

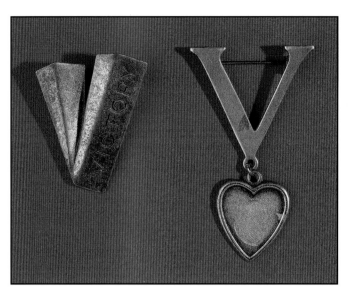

Gold Victory pin. Gold Victory pin with dangling heart emblem. Courtesy of Barbara Trujillo.

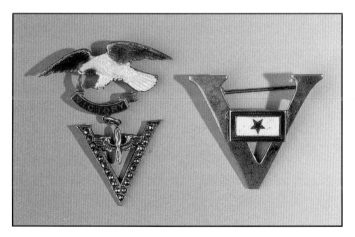

Victory pin with eagle in red, white, and blue colors. Victory pin with plaque in center in red, white, and blue colors. Courtesy of Barbara Trujillo.

Victory pin with "My Son" on top. Courtesy of Barbara Trujillo.

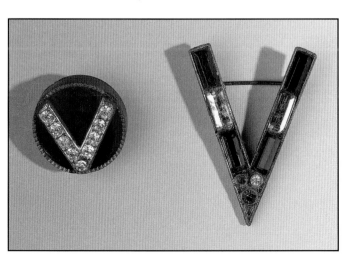

Two Victory pins. Courtesy of Barbara Trujillo.

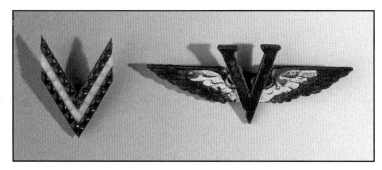

Victory pin in red, white, and blue. Victory pin with spread eagle's wings on either side. Courtesy of Barbara Trujillo.

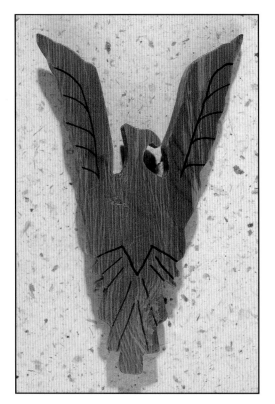

Brown eagle pin of carved wood. Courtesy of Barbara Trujillo.

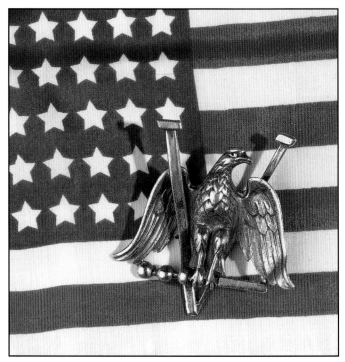

Victory pin with eagle in the center. Courtesy of Barbara Trujillo.

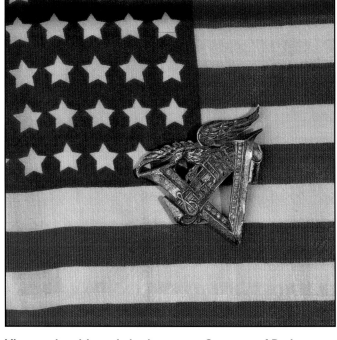

Victory pin with eagle in the center. Courtesy of Barbara Trujillo.

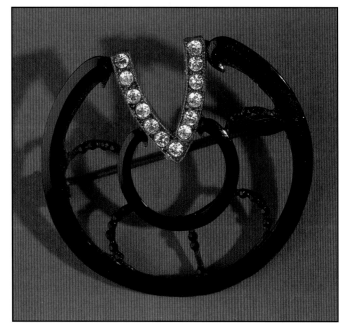

Victory pin. Courtesy of Barbara Trujillo.

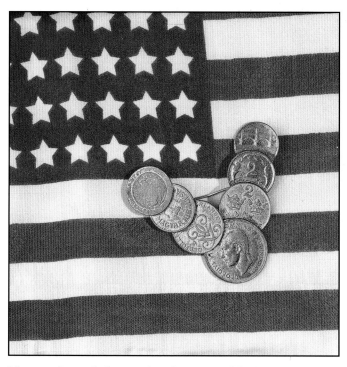

Victory pin made from coins. Courtesy of Barbara Trujillo.

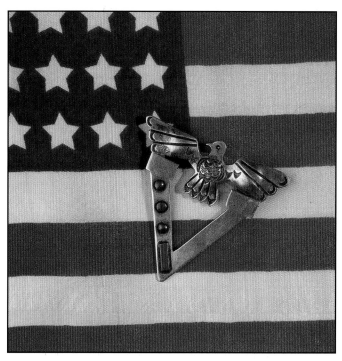

Victory pin with eagle sitting atop and Morse code signal for V. Courtesy of Barbara Trujillo.

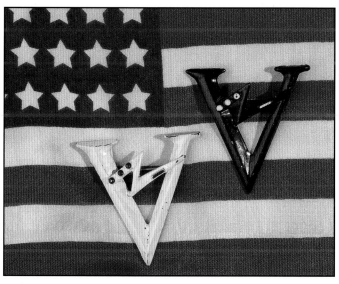

Two Victory pins in white and black enameled metal including the Morse code signal for V. Courtesy of Barbara Trujillo.

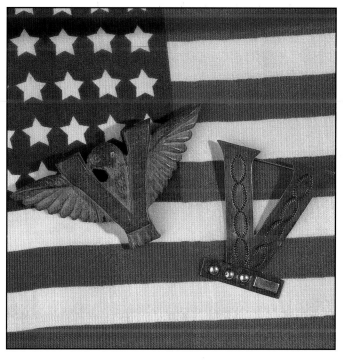

Victory pin with eagle and spread wings. Victory pin with Morse code. Courtesy of Barbara Trujillo.

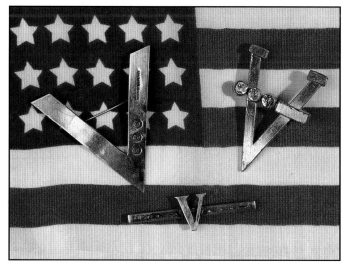

Three Victory pins, all with the Morse code signal for V. Courtesy of Barbara Trujillo.

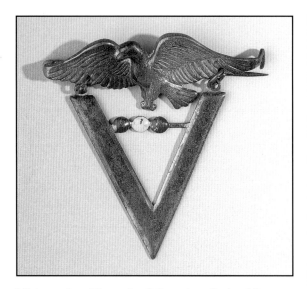

Victory pin with eagle sitting atop. Red, white, and blue colors in the center of V. Courtesy of Barbara Trujillo.

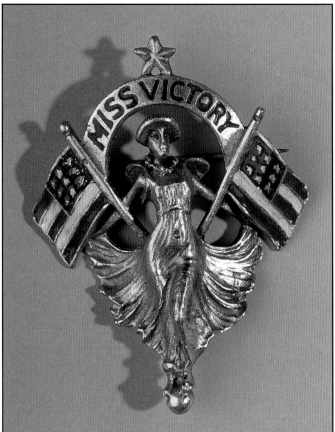

Miss Victory pin. She is holding American flags in both hands.

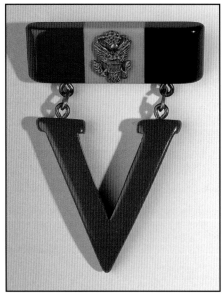

Bakelite Victory pin. 1940s.

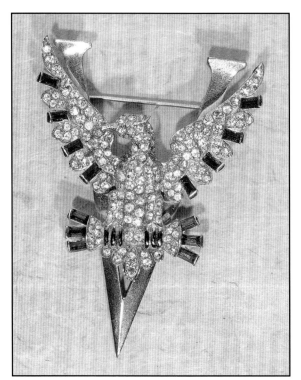

Eagle and V pin with red and blue stones. Signed Mazer. c. 1940s.

Silver pin of a hand, with red, white, and blue bangle bracelets, holding a V for victory. Unmarked. 1940s.

Bibliography

Brunialti, Carla Ginelli and Roberto. *A Tribute to America, Costume Jewelry 1935-1950*. Milan: EDITA, 2002.

Dolan, Maryanne. *Collecting Rhinestone Jewelry*. Florence, Alabama: Books Americana, Inc., 1984.

Ellman, Barbara. *The World of Fashion Jewelry*. Highland Park, Illinois: Aunt Louise Imports, 1986.

Gallina, Jill. *Christmas Pins, Past & Present*. Padukah, Kentucky: Collector Books, 2004.

Kash, Joanne, contributing editor. "V for Victory Dress Pins," *Fashion Accessories*, May, 1991. Collection of Ruth Bon Fleur.

Kelley, Lyngerda and Nancy Schiffer. *Costume Jewelry, The Great Pretenders.* West Chester, Pennsylvania: Schiffer Publishing Ltd., 1987.

Lynnlee, J. L. *All That Glitters*. West Chester, Pennsylvania: Schiffer Publishing Ltd., 1986.

Schiffer, Nancy. *Costume Jewelry, The Fun of Collecting.* West Chester, Pennsylvania: Schiffer Publishing Ltd., 1988.

Shields, Jody. *All That Glitters, The Glory of Costume Jewelry*. New York: Rizzoli International Publications, Inc., 1987.

Snider, Nicholas D. *Antique Sweetheart Jewelry*. Atglen, Pennsylvania: Schiffer Publishing Ltd., 1996.

Snider, Nicholas D. *Sweetheart Jewelry and Collectibles.* Atglen, Pennsylvania: Schiffer Publishing Ltd., 1995.

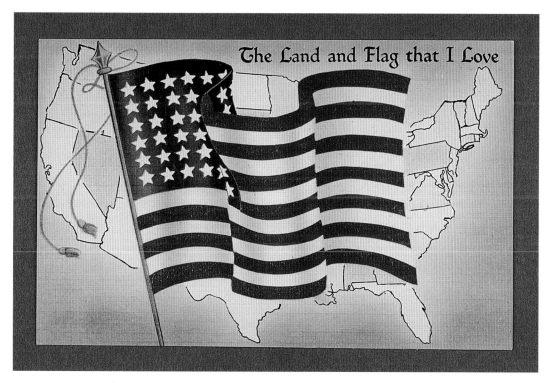

Postcard, 1941. "Tichnor Quality Views" Flag Series No. 10.

Index